PUBLIC HEALTH: PRACTICES, METHODS AND POLICIES

ENVIRONMENTAL HEALTH DISPARITIES

COSTS AND BENEFITS OF BREAKING THE CYCLE

PUBLIC HEALTH: PRACTICES, METHODS AND POLICIES

JOAV MERRICK - SERIES EDITOR –

MEDICAL DIRECTOR, HEALTH SERVICES, DIVISION FOR INTELLECTUAL AND DEVELOPMENTAL DISABILITIES, MINISTRY OF SOCIAL AFFAIRS AND SOCIAL SERVICES, JERUSALEM, ISRAEL

Environment and Public Health: Environmental Health, Law and International Perspectives
I. Leslie Rubin and Joav Merrick (Editors)
2014. ISBN: 978-1-63463-167-9

Health Issues in Diverse Cultures
Cecilia Obeng, Samuel Gyasi Obeng and Joav Merrick (Editors)
2015. ISBN: 978-1-63463-613-1

Tomorrow's Leaders: Service Leadership and Holistic Development in Chinese University Students
Daniel T. L. Shek, Andrew M. H. Siu and Joav Merrick (Editors)
2015. ISBN: 978-1-63321-880-2

Arbovirus: Public Health Experience from Zambia
Seter Siziya, Mazyanga L. Mazaba and Joav Merrick (Editors)
2015. ISBN: 978-1-63463-601-8

Public Health, Social Work and Health Inequalities
Bruce D. Friedman and Joav Merrick (Editors)
2015. ISBN: 978-1-63482-838-3

Smoking and Adolescence: International Public Health Experiences
Mazyanga L Mazaba, Seter Siziya and Joav Merrick (Editors)
2016. ISBN: 978-1-63484-311-9

Environmental Health Disparities: Costs and Benefits of Breaking the Cycle
I Leslie Rubin and Joav Merrick (Editors)
2016. ISBN: 978-1-63484-211-2

PUBLIC HEALTH: PRACTICES, METHODS AND POLICIES

ENVIRONMENTAL HEALTH DISPARITIES

COSTS AND BENEFITS OF BREAKING THE CYCLE

I LESLIE RUBIN
AND
JOAV MERRICK
EDITORS

nova publishers
New York

Library of Congress Cataloging-in-Publication Data

ISBN: 978-1-63484-211-2
Library of Congress Control Number: 2015956240

Published by Nova Science Publishers, Inc. † New York

CONTENTS

PREFACE

This book represents a body of work performed by students from a diverse set of disciplines and a variety of universities. Each project was developed by the students to "break the cycle" of social, economic and environmental health disparities. This book contains the projects from the tenth annual "Break the Cycle" program. "Break the Cycle" projects are designed to raise awareness among students of the reality of environmental health disparities and its impact on the world around them. Although the students may feel daunted by the magnitude of the challenge, they need to know that even the relatively small project they develop can make a big difference and becomes part of an inexorable process towards making the world a better place for all of its citizens. The dictum that "It is not incumbent upon you to finish the task, yet, you are not free to desist from it" empowers the students to take on a challenge for a lifetime. We believe that the lessons learned by the students from their own projects, from working with the other students and from appreciating the difference that each little effort can make, goes significantly towards cultivating our future leaders. They are the people who will carry on the work and make the world a better place.

INTRODUCTION

In: Environmental Health Disparities
Editors: I Leslie Rubin and Joav Merrick
ISBN: 978-1-63484-211-2

Chapter 1

THE COSTS AND BENEFITS OF BREAKING THE CYCLE OF ENVIRONMENTAL HEALTH DISPARITIES

I Leslie Rubin[1-4,*], MD, Robert J Geller[2,5], MD, Kurt Martinuzzi[2,6], MD, Maeve Howett[2,7], APRN, PhD, Benjamin A Gitterman[8], MD, Laura Wells[1,2], MSW, Wayne Garfinkel[9], BSCE, Claire D Coles[10,11], PhD, and Joav Merrick[12-16], MD, MMedSci, DMSc

[1]Innovative Solutions for Disadvantage and Disability, Atlanta, Georgia
[2]Southeast Pediatric Environmental Health Specialty Unit, Emory University, Atlanta, Georgia, US
[3]Department of Pediatrics, Morehouse School of Medicine, Atlanta, Georgia, US
[4]Developmental Pediatric Specialists, Atlanta, Georgia, US
[5]Georgia Poison Center, Grady Health System, Atlanta, Georgia, US
[6]Department of Obstetrics and Gynecology, Emory University School of Medicine, Atlanta, Georgia
[7]Nell Hodgson Woodruff School of Nursing, Emory University, Atlanta, Georgia, US
[8]Departments of Pediatrics and Public Health, George Washington University Schools of Medicine and Public Health and Health Services, General and Community Pediatrics, Children's National Medical Center, Washington DC, US
[9]Children's Environmental Health Coordinator, Atlanta, Georgia
[10]MotherToBaby, Atlanta, Georgia, US
[11]Department of Psychiatry and Behavioral Sciences and Pediatrics, Emory University School of Medicine, Atlanta, Georgia, US
[12]National Institute of Child Health and Human Development, Jerusalem, Israel

* Correspondence: I Leslie Rubin, MD, Associate Professor, Department of Pediatrics, Morehouse School of Medicine and President, Innovative Solutions for Disadvantage and Disability, 750 Hammond Drive, Building 1, Suite 100, Atlanta, GA 30342, United States. E-mail: lrubi01@emory.edu.

[13]Office of the Medical Director, Health Services,
Division for Intellectual and Developmental Disabilities,
Ministry of Social Affairs and Social Services, Jerusalem, Israel
[14]Division of Pediatrics, Hadassah Hebrew University Medical Center,
Mt Scopus Campus, Jerusalem, Israel
[15]Kentucky Children's Hospital, University of Kentucky College of Medicine,
Lexington, Kentucky, US
[16]Center for Human Development, School of Public Health,
Georgia State University, Atlanta, Georgia, US

INTRODUCTION

The social determinants of health are the circumstances in which people are born, grow up, live, work, and age, as well as the systems put in place to deal with illness. These circumstances are in turn shaped by a wider set of forces: economics, social policies, and politics (1).

Healthy People 2020 defines a *health disparity* as "a particular type of health difference that is closely linked with social, economic, and/or environmental disadvantage. Health disparities adversely affect groups of people who have systematically experienced greater obstacles to health based on their racial or ethnic group; religion; socioeconomic status; gender; age; mental health; cognitive, sensory, or physical disability; sexual orientation or gender identity; geographic location; or other characteristics historically linked to discrimination or exclusion" (2).

Healthy People 2020 defines *health equity* as the "attainment of the highest level of health for all people. Achieving health equity, requires valuing everyone equally with focused and ongoing societal efforts to address avoidable inequalities, historical and contemporary injustices, and the elimination of health and health care disparities" (3).

Thus, health inequalities can be defined as differences in health status or in the distribution of health determinants between different population groups. Some health inequalities are attributable to biological variations and others are attributable to the external environment and conditions, mainly outside the control of the individuals concerned. In the first case it may not be possible to change the health determinants and so the health inequalities are unavoidable. In the second, the uneven distribution may be avoidable as well as unjust and unfair, so that the resulting health inequalities also lead to inequity in health (4).

The goals of Healthy People 2020 are:

- Eliminate preventable disease, disability, injury, and premature death.
- Achieve health equity, eliminate disparities, and improve the health of all groups.
- Create social and physical environments that promote good health for all.
- Promote healthy development and healthy behaviors across every stage of life.

They further define environmental determinants of health as follows:

- The *social environment* is the aggregate of social and cultural institutions, norms, patterns, beliefs, and processes that influence the life of an individual or community.
- The *physical environment, comprising both the natural and built environments,* is the structure and function of the environment and how it impacts health.

Children who grow up in circumstances of social and economic disadvantage are more likely to experience multiple stressors in their lives, to have less medical, educational and social support systems in place and to also experience environmental threats from a variety of sources in their homes, their day care centers and schools, their recreational areas and their neighborhoods. These threats include environmental toxins such as outdoor and indoor air pollution, pesticides, secondhand tobacco smoke, waterborne contaminates and specific compounds such as lead and mercury. Evidence linking many medical problems such as asthma, birth defects, and neurodevelopmental disorders to environmental exposures is abundant. Exposures to multiple stressors are also a significant aspect of childhood poverty with far-reaching consequences on biological and psychological regulatory systems resulting in higher incidences of the medical problems which are linked to these exposures (6, 7). We also have evidence of altered brain development in poor children that adversely affects their academic performance and social function (8).

In order to capture these multiple factors and their consequences we conceptualized a cycle of environmental health disparities (see Figure 1) and proceeded to develop a program to explore ways to improve environmental conditions and to reduce these health and functional disparities by "breaking the cycle."

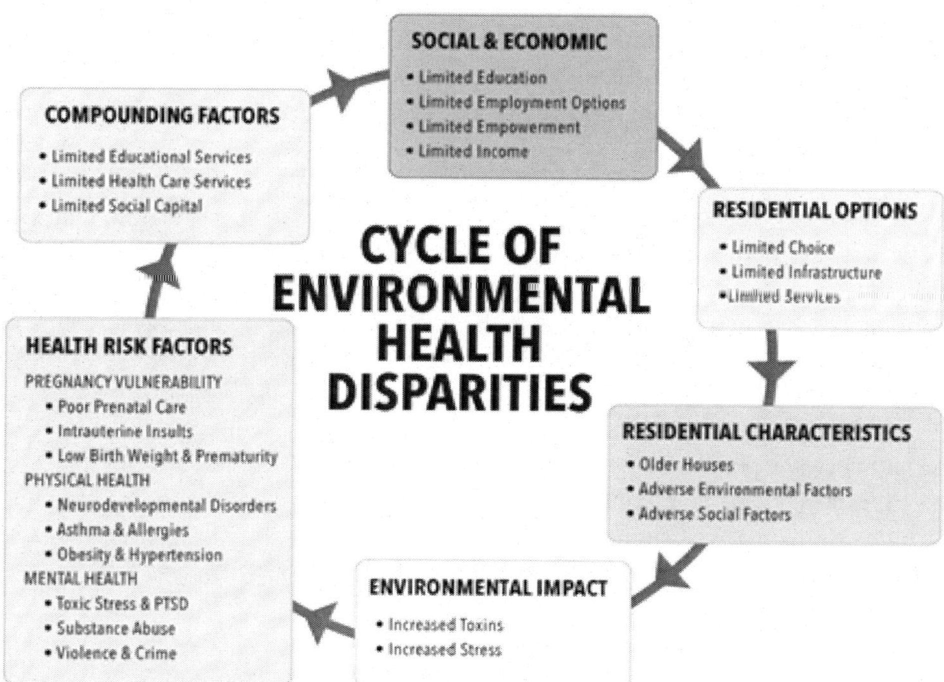

Figure 1. The cycle of environmental health disparities.

Break the cycle

In 2004 we started the "Break the cycle" program to focus on strategies to reduce health disparities. At the same time, we sought to cultivate and inspire a cohort of university students to become aware of the challenges of environmental health disparities in our society and to provide them with the necessary framework and mechanisms to take their youthful ideas, energy and enthusiasm and translate them into working models for reducing health disparities and promoting health equity.

We are pleased to say that after 10 years we have had 10 annual "Break the cycle" programs with over 90 students from 27 different university departments, from nine states in the United States as well as from Latin America, Europe and Africa. The student projects have been published in seven international journals and collected in six books (9).

This publication is of our 10th annual "Break the cycle" program; it represents a diversity of projects and perspectives on the expressions of environmental health disparities in our societies and on some strategies to make a difference in breaking the cycle and offering children opportunities to lead more fulfilling and healthy lives. Each year we identify a theme and try to inform the projects in that idiom and have keynote speakers who address the topic areas. This year our theme was on the cost-benefit of breaking the cycle; in other words, we strive to make a capital investment in the children of today in order to reap dividends to our society in the future. Our feeling was that although the reduction in health disparities and the promotion of health equity do make a difference in the lives of those children in their families who benefit from the projects, we need to show that there are greater changes being wrought and that they have a broader positive impact on our society for the future.

In keeping with our original stated goals, we had anticipated that the projects would make a difference for the particular individuals, their families and their communities where the project took place. However, we also envisioned that the students would be inspired to pursue careers that focused on reducing health disparities and making a bigger difference in the future. Because the students are required to have a mentor at their home university department, we had also hoped that the university faculty mentors would be intrigued enough to add elements of the concept and literature on the subject into their curriculum and thereby promote studies in this field by more of their students – not only the ones in the "Break the cycle" program.

We also anticipated two other elements in the equation, one being that the students would inspire other students in their academic, social and professional circles, and that the interdisciplinary nature of "Break the cycle" program with participation of students at other universities in other cities, states and countries, would be further elucidating and inspiring. A preliminary survey of the students (9) showed that a) they valued guidance in the research process, in the presntaiton at a conference and in the writing of a paper for an academic journal, b) they did perceive a significant benefit in learning about children's environmental health disparities; c) their experiences influenced their professional careers; and d) they did value learning about different perspectives from the other student projects in their particular year.

In choosing the theme of cost-benefit, we wanted to examine more closely the ways in which intervening in a positive way in early childhood could lead to greater benefits for the children as well as for their families, their communities and society at large.

COSTS OF HEALTH DISPARITIES

When we originally conceptualized the cycle of disadvantage and disability in 2004 (see Figure 2) we focused on young women and their children. This was natural from a number of different perspectives; the most significant of which is that it is the women who become pregnant and have children and look after the children who then become the thread of continuity to the next generation. In our model, the adverse social and economic circumstances into which the child is born, predict that the child will be trapped in that cycle and be destined to repeat the pattern unless we do something actively to break the cycle. That had been our mantra with the focus on making a positive difference in the lives of the women and their children. This is an on-going perspective which has sustained the program and the students in the varied ideas and projects that have and will continue to make a difference in breaking the cycle and liberating the women and their children to lead healthier and more successful and productive lives.

While this emphasis seemed natural, it tends to ignore the male children: the boys, the adolescents and the men they will become, who also grow up in the adverse social and economic circumstances, and suffer the effects of poverty and experience the neglect of the neighborhoods, the poor conditions of their schools and less than optimal educational preparation for life's challenges. They tend to have less than inspiring role models of family and friends or 'heroes' that would help them to rise above the day to day pressures and stresses.

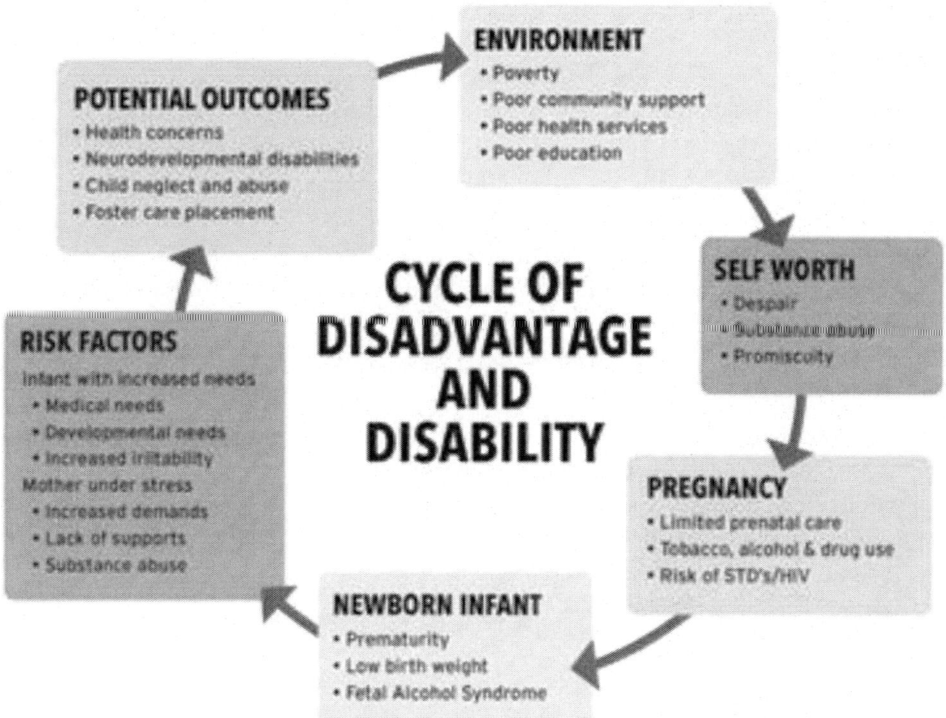

Figure 2. The cycle of disadvantage and disability.

They too, when reaching adolescence and staring at a future which does not hold much promise for advanced education, desirable employment opportunities and limited income, may turn to tobacco, alcohol and other drugs to self-medicate and numb the existential pain, and, for a brief period of time, feel good. Unfortunately these insubstantial and fleeting moments of release from facing a daunting reality and future do not last very long and, without the infrastructural support and encouragement, any notion of a positive future might seem unpromising andbleak.

What then remains for those caught up in this despair is to continue to 'self-medicate' and, unfortunately, become stuck in the vicious cycle where the need for drugs, coupled with unemployment and no financial security can result in selling the drugs to make the money to buy and use the drugs or to steal to support their habit. Either way they risk the chance of being caught, arrested and imprisoned. Obviously this is not universal but the narrative does address and examine the fate of many young men who grow up under these adverse circumstances. Furthermore, their role as fathers is limited. In our original review of the children with cerebral palsy (CP) from poor, minority and underserved communities at the Hughes Spalding Children's Hospital more than 10 years ago, we found that more than 50% of the children with CP were living with single mothers, another 20% with their grandparents and 10% in foster care – only about 20% of the children in the clinic population were living with both biological parents (10). In fact it was extremely rare to see a father or father figure in the many clinics we have had over the more than 15 years of the clinic's existence.

We may then ask: where are they? What has happened to them? The Travis Smiley report on outcomes for young black men in the USA noted the following statistics (11):

- 54% of African Americans graduate from high school, compared to more than three quarters of white and Asian students.
- Nationally, African American male students in grades K-12 were nearly 2½ times as likely to be suspended from school in 2000 as white students.
- In 2007, nearly 6.2 million young people were high school dropouts. Every student who does not complete high school costs our society an estimated $260,000 in lost earnings, taxes, and productivity.
- On average, African American twelfth-grade students read at the same level as white eighth-grade students.
- The twelfth-grade reading scores of African American males were significantly lower than those for men and women across every other racial and ethnic group.
- Only 14% of African American eighth graders score at or above the proficient level. These results reveal that millions of young people cannot understand or evaluate text, provide relevant details, or support inferences about the written documents they read.
- The majority of the 2.3 million people incarcerated in U.S. prisons and jails are people of color, people with mental health issues and drug addiction, people with low levels of educational attainment, and people with a history of unemployment or underemployment.

In the documentary film "Waiting for Superman" there is a vivid cartoon illustrating the commentary that it costs approximately $30,000 a year for people to be in prison, and that, if this money would be invested in early childhood education, not only would this money be saved, but that the children would grow up to be contributing members of society (12). Interestingly, a review of annual costs of imprisonment per inmate in 2010 varied from a low of about $14,000 in Indiana and Kentucky to a high of about $60,000 in New York. (13) The Department of Justice, Bureau of Prisons gives an average figure of $28,893.40/inmate for 2011 (14). Another report from the New York City Independent Budget Office states that 'the average annual cost per inmate in 2012 was $167,731, which probably includes many other costs associated with imprisonment (15) They also report that of the inmates in 2012, 57 percent were black, 33 percent Hispanic, 7 percent white, 1 percent Asian, and the rest 'other or unknown', and 97% were male. These statistics certainly paint a very grim picture.

The sad reality is that the USA has the highest incarceration rate in the world at 716 per 100,000 population, in the Russian Federation there are 475/100,000, and in countries of Western Europe the rates are substantially less than 100 per 100,000 population! (16) While the prison population has grown exponentially in the USA since the 1980's so have the costs to the national and state budgets grown.

In California in 2010, where the cost per inmate was about $47,000 per year, the total cost of prisons is almost $8 billion/year. (13). In the California Governor's Budget of 2015-2016 the costs for the California Department of Corrections and Rehabilitation has risen of the past years to $10.2 billion (9.0% of the budget) while the budget allocation for Human Services is 7.8 billion (6.9% of the budget) and that for Higher Education is just $14billion (12.4% of the budget). More will be spent on correction than on support to prevent the need for correction. It is gratifying to see that the budget for higher education is higher than that for corrections but not by much! (17).

Once again it is critical to point out that the costs of imprisonment represent a significant loss to society, payments that have no dividends. The sad reality is that prisons do more harm than good to individuals, their families and to society. In his Walter C Reckless memorial lecture 'Thinking about prison and its impact in the twenty-first century' Marc Mauer reviewed the negative impact of incarceration, he noted that individuals returning from prison have difficulty getting jobs, earning money and regaining self-respect. In addition, their families and communities suffer an emotional and financial toll during the period of incarceration, as well as after release, and the individuals have difficulty reintegrating into society. The high incarceration rate reflects on our society, and comes at a high cost financially, morally and to our democratic identity (18).

As a corollary, if we can invest in the education and moral upbringing of children, we are more likely to see them become successful academically, socially and economically. Then, not only will they not be a drain on taxpayers' funds, but they will be actively contributing to the tax revenue by working and earning good money and benefiting all of society financially and in many other ways.

Our investments in the education process will then have paid great dividends and the benefits to the individual and to society will have far outweighed the costs. Not only that, but by successfully breaking the negative cycle, we will have created a positive one because their children will in turn benefit and prosper and be more likely continue the positive cycle.

EARLY CHILDHOOD EDUCATION

In the early 1960's the "Perry preschool program" was started at the Perry Elementary School in Ypsilanti Michigan focusing on children who were living in circumstances of social and economic disadvantage who had a low IQ. Beginning at age 3 years and lasting 2 years, treatment consisted of a 2.5-hour preschool program on weekdays during the school year, supplemented by weekly home visits by teachers. Follow-up interviews were conducted when participants were approximately 15, 19, 27, and 40 years old. At these interviews, participants provided detailed information about their life-cycle trajectories including schooling, economic activity, marital life, child rearing, and incarceration.

In addition, Perry researchers collected administrative data in the form of school records, police and court records, and records on welfare participation. In 2010, the Nobel laureate, James Heckman and his colleagues reviewed the outcome data on the study and concluded that for the undiscounted year-2006 dollars, cost of the program per child was $17,759. The return on investment looking at education, employment and earnings, reduction in criminal activity, increase tax payments, reduction on welfare dependence, and excluding benefits from improvements in health status was between 7-10%, which is a substantial return on investment. Of note, they comment that 'benefits from improvements in health and the well-being of future generations are not estimated due to data limitations.' They thus point out that their results did not take into consideration the longer term benefits of stability and security for the children thereby reaching into the future and breaking the cycle (19).

ELEMENTARY SCHOOL EDUCATION

In the mid 1980's, the STAR Program (The Student/Teacher Achievement Ratio) was launched at 79 schools across Tennessee. A total of 11,571 students and their teachers in grades K–3 were randomly assigned to small class sizes of about 15 students per class, or to larger classes of about 22 students per classroom. The researchers then looked at the students at age 27 years and examined outcome measures such as college attendance, earnings, retirement savings, home ownership, and marriage (20). They noted that a number of long-term outcomes were significantly associated with Kindergarten test scores such as earnings, college attendance rates, quality of college attended, home ownership, and 401(k) savings. Students assigned to small classes were more likely to be enrolled in college at age 20 years. These students went on to have higher rates of home ownership, larger 401(k) savings, increased mobility, were more likely to graduate from college and were more likely to be married. Students assigned to teachers with 10 or more years of experience and were in classes with high achieving students, had occupations with enhanced earning. Of note is that the impact of class size on test scores 'faded out' by 8th grade but that the Kindergarten class quality continued to have a significant impact on non-cognitive measures in 4th and 8th grade such as effort, initiative, and lack of disruptive behavior. In addition, they found that these elements correlated with significantly higher earnings, perhaps the behavior characteristics were more desirable in the labor market. Overall therefore, these advantages of small classroom size, teacher experience, positive peer groups, and 'quality' of the classroom, predicted not only enhanced earning potential but college attendance, marital status, and savings for the future in a 401(k) – this being another element in the breaking of the cycle towards a more positive future for their children and for society at large. Once again, the investment in quality education for children in Kindergarten and the early grades does make a difference in the long term outcome for children as they grow into adulthood and take responsibility for their own actions and plan for the future in caring for and about their children, their communities and society.

VALUE ADDED TEACHERS

In 2011, Chetty et al. (21), economists at Harvard and Columbia Universities, reviewed data on 2.5 million school children from 3rd to 8th grade and linked them to tax records and other long term outcome data. They were looking to see whether exposure of students to a Value Added Teacher made a difference to the child in the long term. A teacher's "value-added" (VA) status is defined as the average test-score gain for his or her students, adjusted for differences across classrooms in student characteristics. When a high VA teacher (top 5%) enters a school, the end-of-school-year test scores in the grade he or she teaches, rise immediately. Students assigned to high-VA teachers are more likely to attend college, attend higher- ranked colleges, earn higher salaries, live in a higher socioeconomic status (SES) neighborhoods, and save more for retirement. They are also less likely to have children as teenagers. Again, the impact of a positive intervention will have a beneficial effect not only on the individual, but on that individual's children as well as on society. From a financial and cost-benefit perspective, Chetty et al. note that, 'having such a teacher for one year raises a child's cumulative lifetime income by $80,000 (equivalent to $14,500 in present value at age 12 with a 5% interest rate). They further extrapolate that the earnings gains from replacing a low value-added (bottom 5%) teacher with one of average quality grow as more data are used to estimate the benefits of VA teachers. Discounting future earnings gains to present value, the gains are $270,000 with 3 years of data. If future earnings are not discounted, cumulative earnings gains surpass $1.4 million per class (22)'.

MAKING A DIFFERENCE IN THE SCHOOL

Schools in low income communities are often in poor condition. Old buildings with poor air control systems may result in increased pollution from sources such as art supplies and laboratory activities, temperature control and humidity, moisture and spills, inadequate ventilation, poor housekeeping and maintenance operations and outdoor pesticide use.

Studies have demonstrated that lighting, ventilation, temperature control and indoor air quality affect health and performance. Indoor air quality problems can result in school absences linked to asthma, allergies and respiratory diseases. According to the Centers for Disease Control and Prevention (CDC), asthma related illness is one of the leading causes of school absenteeism, accounting for over 10 million missed school days per year (23). Students who miss more school score lower on standardized tests and are more likely to drop out before graduating from high school.

Improving management of asthma can significantly reduce episodes of asthma that reduce school attendance, but, it is critical to reduce the environmental factors that trigger asthmatic attacks such as the poor air quality in older and dilapidated schools. Schools should be designed, built and maintained to minimize and control sources of pollution, provide adequate exhaust and outdoor air ventilation, and supply proper temperature and humidity conditions. School systems can take advantage of available programs such as EPA's Indoor Air Quality Tools for Schools Program to improve and maintain optimum conditions (24).

With improved environmental conditions in schools, chidlren with asthma will be less likely to experience asthmatic episodes and less likely to miss days at school and more likely to keep up with school work and graduate. Improved environmental conditions in schools will likewise improve the health and well-being of everyone in the school and with improved sense of well-being comes improved function and with improved function comes improved likelihood of success.

MAKING A DIFFERENCE IN NEIGHBORHOODS

Moving to opportunity (MTO) was a large HUD-funded demonstration program in 1994 involving 4,600 low income families from poor neighborhoods. The MTO program set up 3 groups within these families - one group was offered a housing voucher that could only be used to move from their high-poverty neighborhood to a low-poverty neighborhood, a second group was offered a traditional Section 8 housing voucher, and a control group who remained in place (25). The anticipated outcome was that the families who moved would be better off physically, mentally, socially and financially. The families were evaluated at intervals from 2 years after the move until recently after 18 years.

Interestingly, the benefits seemed to change over time; in the early years of the move there appeared to be benefits to health (26), behavior and education (27), however, some of the benefits disappeared in later evaluations leading to confusion and disappointment that the experiment had been a failure (28). Recently however, the economist, Rav Chettey of Harvard University and his colleagues in a National Bureau of Economic Research working paper 15-18 years after the move, used federal tax records looking at the adults who moved as children found that the incomes of those in their mid-20's was raised by 31% (29). What was striking however, was that these outcomes were only for the children who moved before the age of 13 years and not after. This raises two important issues: one that neighborhood matters to children and two, that it makes a big difference if you start at a young age. This exemplifies the cost benefit of "early intervention" in the long term that benefits not only the individual but also the family, the neighborhood, the community and all of society.

MAKING A DIFFERENCE ACROSS GENERATIONS

Epigenetic data provides a basis for demonstrating that the effect of biosocial behaviors can have an impact across generations. In their landmark study on maternal grooming behavior of rats, researchers at McGill University found that some rats would be more maternal in licking and grooming their pups to a greater degree while others were somewhat neglectful and did not lick or groom their pups much. The pups who were nurtured by licking and grooming turned out to be less anxious and had a low stress response, while the pups who had been neglected, who had not been licked and groomed, tended to be more anxious and had a higher stress response. When these pups were followed into their next generation, the mothers, who as pups, had been licked and groomed, would go on to lick and groom their own pups, while the mothers who had not been nurtured as pups, went on to neglect their offspring much as they had been neglected. If however, the pups born to neglectful mothers were given to the nurturing mothers who would lick and groom them; those pups when they grew up would become nurturing mothers, much as they had been treated as pups. The message is clear – we can make a difference where we had not realized before. The transgenerational behavior patterns were not as much genetically determined but were epigenetic, in that the genes could be modified and activated by appropriate stimuli with a positive outcome for the individual rats as well as for their offspring into future generations (30).

The stress patterns of the neglected rat pups could be compared to the toxic stress phenomenon that plays out in children who had repeated adverse childhood experiences (31). These children go on to developing unhealthy behaviors and are more likely to use tobacco, alcohol or other drugs, and other risk taking behaviors, with difficulty maintaining supportive social networks and are at risk for school failure, gang membership, unemployment, poverty, homelessness, violent crime, incarceration, and becoming single parents. Furthermore, adults in this high-risk group who become parents themselves, are less likely to be able to provide the kind of stable and supportive family relationships that are needed to protect their children from the damages of toxic stress. This intergenerational cycle of significant adversity, with its predictable repetition of limited educational achievement and poor health, is mediated, at least in part, by the social inequalities and disrupted social networks that contribute to fragile families and parenting difficulties.

Thus the stories of children who are neglected and experience adverse life events repeatedly have the same physiological mechanisms as the epigenetic studies cited above. It follows therefore, that if we can prevent children from having these adverse experiences and provide for them the nurturing they need to develop healthy physiological and behavioral coping mechanisms, we will certainly break the cycle and these children will be more likely to go on to attend good schools.

COST BENEFIT OF MAKING A DIFFERENCE

Professor James Heckman, Nobel laureate in economics, has focused his knowledge, talents and skills on examining the impact of poverty on the developing child and the implications for the economics of our society (32). He links poverty with limited nurturing, poor academic performance, limited literacy, limited employment opportunities and ultimate involvement in the criminal justice system, which sounds very much like our cycle of disadvantage and disability concept. He further maintains that it is not merely the lack of financial resources, that takes its toll on the cognitive skills of the child, but the lack of cognitive and non-cognitive stimulation given to young children by their mothers and their families. As an economist he sees this as a serious issue that affects our entire society in that the cost of letting children suffer from lack of support and education takes a toll, not only on the child and family, but on the economy of a society. By his calculation the cost of crime in American society is in the trillions of dollars which translates in a per capita cost of at least several thousand dollars a year.

He maintains that early intervention, as early as possible is the answer, while the brain is still young and ready to be wired for success. He cites as an example data from the Perry Preschool Program (19) and concludes that the benefits accrued as a result of higher earnings, savings in welfare and reduced costs of crime are at $8.74 to $1 on investment. He even feels that this project did not look at children young enough (they were 3-4years of age) and that an even earlier start and earlier intervention would likely result in even greater savings in human lives as well as in dollars and that the society at large will benefit. His plea is for early intervention and early education not only because it makes sound physiological, psychological and sociological sense but because it makes sound economic sense. These are his words on his website where he urges to invest in early childhood development to reduce deficits and strengthen the economy (33):

> "The highest rate of return in early childhood development comes from investing as early as possible, from birth through age five, in disadvantaged families. Starting at age three or four is too little too late, as it fails to recognize that skills beget skills in a complementary and dynamic way. Efforts should focus on the first years for the greatest efficiency and effectiveness. The best investment is in quality early childhood development from birth to five for disadvantaged children and their families."

See Figure 3 for his schematic on costs and benefits at the difference chronological ages (32). Heckman calculates that the greater investment in the preschool age group – the younger the better – yields the greatest cost-benefit, while investments in schools and post schools, while unquestionable important, have much lower yields unless the child has been primed at a preschool age.

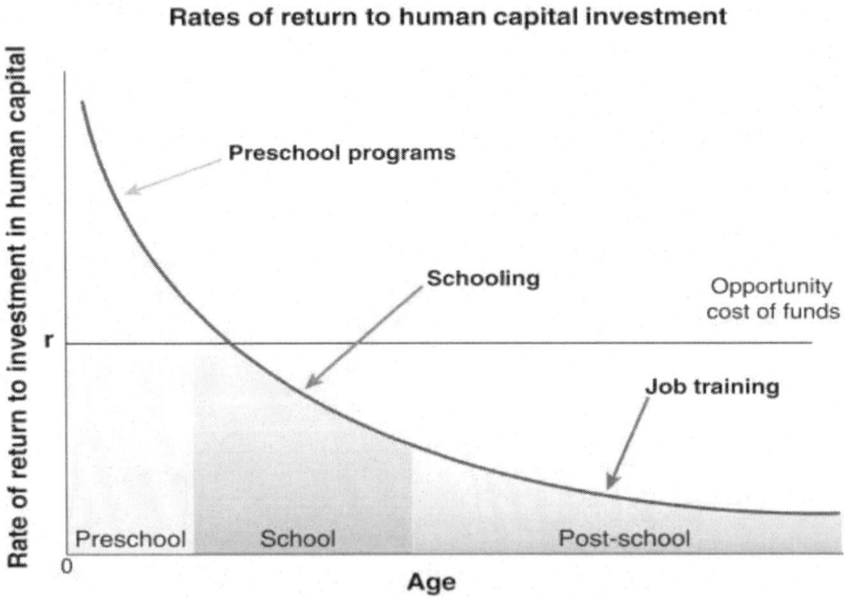

Figure 3. Rates of return to human capital investment in disadvantaged children (32).

CONCLUSION

Health disparities and health inequities are prevalent in all societies and in all sectors of society. They are part of the reality of life and its political, social, economic and environmental determinants that play out in a multilayered dynamic. Even though the idea of health equity for all children is an ideal which may not necessarily be achievable, it should nonetheless be the goal to which we aspire. The big and small projects that have been described in this paper are all part of the panorama; each one of them looks at a different facet of the challenge and a different facet of the potential solution. And, even though we may not necessarily be able to accomplish our goal, we are absolutely obligated to continue to make a positive difference in breaking the cycle because ultimately we all benefit – the children, their families, their communities and society benefit physically, emotionally, socially, financially and morally. Evidence strongly points to the need to act early – early intervention can never be too early to reap maximum benefit; the later the intervention, the greater cost and the smaller the benefit (see Figure 3).

As has been demonstrated and as has been stated several times in this paper, it is critical to intervene early in the life of a child if one wants to have the greatest beneficial impact. For the rat pups it is in the immediate newborn period during nursing – licking and grooming. For infants and children it is having supportive and loving parents in a loving, stable and secure home. For children it is to have a good education in a safe and healthy school with good teachers, and for adolescents and families it is to live in safe and secure neighborhoods with strong and supportive communities to be there for each other in times of need. If we want to make the biggest impact on the newborn infant and young child, we need to reach the parents before they become parents, when they are teenagers thinking about their futures, we need to help them to find their senghts and cultivate their sense of a positive future. It is all in the cycle, in changing the the trajectory.

Ultimately we also need to recognize that each individual has the potential to change for the better, some on their own with sheer determination and a modicum of support and opportunity, while others may require more support and assistance. It is our responsibility to attempt to make a difference for all vulnerable children, for it is said that: if you save the life of one child, it is as if you are saving the world. In the context of our cycle model, it is to change it from one of disadvantage and disability, to one of ability and advantage.

ACKNOWLEDGMENTS

The US Environmental Protection Agency (EPA) supports the PEHSU by providing partial funding to ATSDR under Inter-Agency Agreement number DW-75-95877701. Neither EPA nor ATSDR endorse the purchase of any commercial products or services mentioned in PEHSU publications.

REFERENCES

[1] Center for Disease Control and Prevention. Social determinants of health. URL: http://www.cdc.gov/nchhstp/socialdeterminants/index.html.

[2] Healthy People 2020. The Secretary's Advisory Committee on National Health Promotion and Disease Prevention Objectives for 2020. Phase 1 report October 8, 2008. URL: http://www.healthypeople.gov/sites/default/files/PhaseI_0.pdf.

[3] Healthy People 2020. Office of Disease Prevention and Health Promotion: Healthy people 2020. URL: http://www.healthypeople.gov/2020/about/foundation-health-measures/Disparities.

[4] World Health Organization. Glossary of terms. URL: http://www.who.int/hia/about/glos/en/index1.html.

[5] Healthy People 2020. Secretary's Advisory Committee on National Health Promotion and Disease Prevention Objectives for 2020. US Department of Health and Human Services. July 26, 2010. URL: http://www.healthypeople.gov/2010/hp2020/advisory/societaldeterminantshealth.htm.

[6] Evans H, Kim P. Childhood poverty, chronic stress, and coping. Child Dev Perspect 2013;7:43-48.

[7] Kim P, Neuendorf C, Bianco H, Evans GW. Exposure to childhood poverty and mental health symptomatology in adolescence: A role of coping strategies. Stress Health 2015 Aug 3. doi: 10.1002/smi.2646.

[8] Hair NL, Hanson JL, Wolfe BL, Pollak SD. Association of Child Poverty, Brain Development, and Academic Achievement. JAMA Pediatr. 2015 Jul 20. doi: 10.1001/jamapediatrics.

[9] Rubin IL, Oves D, Nodvin J, Geller RJ, Howett M, Martinuzzi K, Gitterman BA, Wells L, Merrick J. Break the cycle: Survey of past students, 2005-2011 student Survey. Int J Child Health Hum Dev 2016;9(4), in press.

[10] Rubin IL, Geller RJ, Nodvin J,, Ace K, Merrick J. Break the cycle to improve health and developmental outcomes for all children. Int J Child Adolesc Health 2009;2:265-72.

[11] Thompson T. Fact sheet: Outcomes for young Black men. Episode 5 Travis Smiley reports. URL: http://www.pbs.org/wnet/tavissmiley/tsr/too-important-to-fail/fact-sheet-outcomes-for-young-black-men/.

[12] Guggenheim D. Waiting for "Superman": How we can save America's failing public schools, 2010. URL: http://www.takepart.com/waiting-for-superman.

[13] Henrichson C, Delaney R. The price of prisons. What incarceration costs taxpayers. New York: Vera Institute of Justice, 2012.

[14] Department of Justice. Annual determination of average cost of incarceration. Federal Register 2013;78(52):16711.

[15] New York City Independent Budget Office. New York City by the Numbers, 2014. URL: http://ibo.nyc.ny.us/cgi-park2/?cat=21.

[16] Walmsley R. International Center for Prison Studies, World Population List 10th Edition. International Centre for Prison Studies, 2013. URL: http://www.prisonstudies.org/sites/default/files/resources/downloads/wppl_10.pdf.

[17] Brown Jr EG. 2015-2016 State of California Budget, 2015. URL: http://www.ebudget.ca.gov/2015-16/pdf/BudgetSummary/FullBudgetSummary.pdf.

[18] Mauer M. Thinking about prison and its impact in the twenty-first century: Walter C Reckless memorial lecture. Ohio State J Crim Law 2005;2:607-18.

[19] Heckman JJ. Moon SH, Pinto R, Savelyev P, Yavitz A. A new cost-benefit and rate of return analysis for the Perry Preschool Program: A summary. Bonn: IZA Policy Papers 17, Institute for the Study of Labor (IZA), 2010.

[20] Chetty R, Friedman JN, Hilger N, Saez E, Schanzenbach D, Yagan D. How does your kindergarten classroom affect your earnings? Evidence from Project STAR. Quart J Econ 2011;126(4):1593-1660.

[21] Chetty R, Friedman JN, Rockoff JE. The long-term impacts of teachers: Teacher value-added and student outcomes in adulthood. Cambridge, MA: National Bureau of Economic Research, 2011, Revised 2012.

[22] Chetty R, Friedman JN, Rockoff JE. Measuring the impacts of teachers II: Teacher value-added and student outcomes in adulthood. Am Econ Rev 2014;104(9):2633-79.

[23] Meng Y, Babey SH, Wolstein J. Asthma-related school absenteeism and school concentration of low-income students in California. Prev Chronic Dis 2012;9:110312.

[24] EPA indoor air quality tools for schools program. URL: http://www.efc.gwu.edu/wp-content/uploads/2014/05/EPA_Indoor-air-quality-tools-for-schools-program.pdf.

[25] Brennan B, Sciandra M. History of MTO. Moving to opportunity research. URL: http://www.nber.org/mtopublic/history.htm.

[26] Ludwig J, Sanbonmatsu L, Gennetian L, Adam E, Duncan GJ, Katz LF, et al. Neighborhoods, obesity, and diabetes: A randomized social experiment. N Engl J Med 2011;365:1509-19.

[27] Moving to opportunity (MTO) for fair housing demonstration program. URL: http://www.nber.org/mtopublic/.

[28] Rothwell J. Sociology's revenge: Moving to opportunity (MTO) revisited. Brookings, 2015. URL: http://www.brookings.edu/blogs/social-mobility-memos/posts/2015/05/06-moving-to-opportunity-revisited-rothwell 29. Chetty R, Hendren N. The impacts of neighborhoods on intergenerational mobility: Childhood exposure effects and county-level estimates. Working paper, 2015. URL: http://www.equality-of-opportunity.org/images/nbhds_paper.pdf.

[29] Weaver IC, Cervoni N, Champagne FA, D'Alessio AC, Sharma S, Seckl JR, et al. Epigenetic programming by maternal behavior. Nat Neurosci 2004;7(8):847-54.

[30] Shonkoff JP, Garner AS, Committee on Psychological Aspects of Child and Family Health, Committee on Early Childhood, Adoption, and Dependent Care, and Section on Developmental and Behavioral Pediatrics. The lifelong effects of early childhood adversity and toxic stress. Pediatrics 2012;129(1):e232-46.

[31] Heckman JJ, Skill formation and the economics of investing in disadvantaged children. Science 2006;312:1900-2.

[32] Heckman JJ. Invest in early childhood development: Reduce deficits, strengthen the economy, 2012, URL: http://heckmanequation.org/content/resource/invest-early-childhood-development-reduce-deficits-strengthen-economy.

SECTION ONE: COMMUNITY CHARACTERISTICS

In: Environmental Health Disparities
Editors: I Leslie Rubin and Joav Merrick
ISBN: 978-1-63484-211-2

Chapter 2

ENVIRONMENTAL RISK FACTORS AND MALNUTRITION IN CHILDREN UNDER THE AGE OF FIVE LIVING IN ZAMBIA

Chalwe Chanda*[*]*, BScEH,
and Nosiku S Munyinda, BScNRM, MScEnvEng
Environmental Health Unit, Department of Public Health,
School of Medicine, The University of Zambia, Lusaka, Zambia

More than three million children under the age of five years die each year from environment-related conditions. In many countries in Africa, these factors are related to malnutrition, lack of access to clean water, and the risk of infections. Methods: We conducted a cross-sectional, household study in the Chipata compound of the Lusaka District, Zambia, over a 4-week period in early 2015. The study population included all mothers with children aged 6 months to 59 months obtaining health services from the Chipata First Level Hospital. Systematic random sampling guided the recruitment. We investigated the nutrition status of the children, maternal factors, and environmental factors such as housing and sanitation. Results: We found that children age under five years in Chipata Compound of Lusaka City lived in a low income unplanned community, with low cost housing, and were exposed to highly unsanitary conditions. We found that children born of teenage mothers were not at a higher risk of being malnourished than those born from older mothers. Housing status showed a highly significant association with nutrition status of the child (p = 0.01). However, sanitation facility, source of drinking water, and availability of waste collection services showed a relatively weaker relationship with nutrition in children. With the unimproved pit latrine as the most common sanitary facility, contamination of groundwater is highly plausible. Further, the low income housing contributes to the high contamination of drinking water sources, resulting in diarrhoeal infections, and eventual malnourishment in the under-five child.

[*] Correspondence: Chalwe Chanda, BScEH, Environmental Health Unit, Department of Public Health, The University of Zambia, School of Medicine, POBox 50110, Lusaka, Zambia. E-mail: blesschanda88@yahoo.com.

INTRODUCTION

The World Health Organization estimates that 50% of malnutrition is related to the consumption of unsafe water, inadequate sanitation, and poor hygiene, which results in repeated bouts of diarrhoea and intestinal worm infection (1). More than three million children under the age of five years die annually from environment-related causes. Individuals who live in deprived areas with poor sanitation, inadequate hygiene, and unsafe drinking water are exposed to enteric pathogens which cause diarrheal illnesses (2). Intestinal worms infect over 85% of children in the developing world, leading to malnutrition, anaemia, and retarded growth (3). In addition to infection, risk factors for malnutrition include inadequate dietary intake and limited access to maternal and child healthcare. Breast feeding and good basic hygiene practices such as hand washing decrease the risk of infection and hence the risk for malnutrition (4).

Neonates are born with passive immunity acquired from their mothers. As this immunity wanes, infections increase between the ages of six to 24 months of life. Malnutrition and anaemia follows and often cannot be fully reversed (5, 6). Because the causes of malnutrition are multi-factorial, successful intervention must occur at both the community and household level (5).

In recent decades, adolescent pregnancy has become an important health issue in many countries, both developed and developing countries. Undernourished girls have a greater likelihood of becoming undernourished mothers, who in turn have a greater chance of giving birth to low-birth-weight babies (7). In a cohort study carried out in a densely populated section of Freetown, Sierra Leone (8), a strong positive correlation was discovered between older age of the mothers and improved nutritional status of the child. Children of younger mothers had higher mortality rates, due to increased malnutrition, measles and diarrheal diseases, the three major disease conditions associated with under-five mortality.

In a study conducted to assess the nutritional status and feeding practices of children under the age of 5 years among the pastoral communities of Simanjiro District, northern Tanzania, an educated mother was less likely to have an undernourished child, while a teenage mother was more likely to have an undernourished child (9).

The Zambia Bureau of Statistics (10) has shown that education attainment has a strong effect on nutrition. Similarly, the United States Agency for International Development (USAID) (11) noted that mothers' education was related to knowledge of good childcare practices, including appropriate meals to be given to infants, and diagnosis and treatment of common illnesses. In India, educated mothers were found to be more likely to acquire knowledge or to adopt new ideas related to nutrition and health issues than were less-educated mothers (12). Other factors that influence food intake include health status, food taboos, and personal choice (13).

OUR STUDY

We conducted a cross-sectional, household study in the Chipata compound of the Lusaka District over a 4-week period in early 2015. Chipata covers some 1,000 hectares and has a population of approximately 45,000 (about 10,000 households). The Chipata compound is a squatter settlement and was declared "an improvement area" under the Zambia Housing (Statutory and Improvement Area) Act. The community considered water supply to be its highest priority need. The source population for study was all mothers with children aged 6 months to 59 months obtaining health services from the Chipata First Level Hospital. Systematic random sampling guided the recruitment.

The data collection techniques used were researcher-administered questionnaires and review of children's under-five cards. An under-five card is maintained for every child. Each time a mother makes a monthly visit to a hospital or clinic, the weight of the child is recorded to show the growth curve for the child. The card also has the child's health history and immunization details. The growth regions on the card are standardized using WHO classifications. We also surveyed the housing, sanitation and access to drinking water as well as access to health care.

Table 1. Socio demographic characteristics of the respondents, n = 88

Variable	Frequency	Percentage (%)
Mother age		
13 years – 19 years	19	21.6
20 years – 27 years	69	78.4
Marital status		
Single	11	12.5
Married	73	83.0
Divorced	3	3.4
Widowed	1	1.1
Mothers educational status		
No form of education	3	3.4
Primary	36	40.9
Secondary	46	52.3
Tertiary	3	3.4
Child sex		
Female	35	39.8
Male	53	60.2
Children age in months		
6 months - 23 months	70	79.5
24 months - 59 months	18	20.5
Number of children per mother		
1 – 3 children	73	83.0
4 and above	15	17.0
Number of household members		
Between 1 and 5	68	77.3
Between 6 and 10	19	21.6
Above 10	1	1.1
Number of rooms		
1 – 3 rooms	79	89.8
4 and above	9	10.2
Housing status		
Low income housing	82	93.2
Medium income housing	6	6.8
Total	**88**	**100.0**

Data was analysed using the statistical package SPSS. To assess the associations, the dependent variable (nutrition status) was compared with the independent variables in cross tabulations. Chi Square tests were used to assess the strength of the associations.

FINDINGS

Mothers participating in this study were 21.6% of teen age and 78.4% aged 20 years and over (see Table 1). This age distribution is similar to that found in the 2007 Zambia Demographic Health Survey (ZDHS), a nationally representative survey of 7,146 women aged 15-49 years, which revealed that about 28% (2,000) of women aged 15-19 years had begun childbearing.

In this study, 40.9% had completed primary education, 52.3% secondary education, 3.4% tertiary education, while 3.4% had not received any formal education.

Of the 88 children under the age of five, 60.2% were male and 39.8% were female. 31.8% of the children were underweight and 18.2% had moderate to severe acute malnutrition. More girls (23.9%) were found to be underweight than boys (8.0%) ($p = 0.053$). Of children born to teenage mothers, 4.5% were underweight and 3.4% had moderate to severe acute malnourishment. There was no association between the mother's age at the child's birth and incidence of being underweight ($p = 0.197$) or having severe acute malnourishment. ($p = 0.675$).

Most of the children (79.5%) ranged in age from 6-23 months, with the remaining 20.5% of the children inages 24-59 months (see Table 1). The incidence of moderate to severe acute malnutrition was statistically significantly greater in the younger children ($p = 0.025$).

The highest proportion of mothers (93.2%) were living in low cost houses. Most households had 1-5 members (77.3%); 21.6% of households were 6-10 in size and only 1.1% of households had 10 or more members. Housing status was a highly significant risk factor for severe acute malnutrition ($p = 0.001$) but not associated with children being underweight; children who lived in overcrowded houses were at a high risk of being wasted. Spouse employment status, monthly income, marital status, and paternal support did not affect the incidence of children who were underweight or had severe acute malnutrition. Over 70% of the mothers recruited were married; those single or divorced received support from their families.

Zambia is one of the world's poorest countries with per capita annual income of $395. Due to unemployment and under-employment 70% of Zambians live in abject poverty (21). This study revealed that the highest proportion of respondents (47.7%) earned between 200 Zambian Kwacha and 500 Zambian Kwacha, 35.5% earned slightly above 500 Zambian Kwacha, 4.5% earned below 200 Zambian Kwacha, while 12.5% had no form of employment and depended on spouses or parents (see Table 2). This meant that the highest proportion of respondents lived on between $1 and $2 per day. Only 13.6% of study participants had formal employment; those without formal employment or dependent on parental support comprised 86.4%. This finding was similar to the national survey (Zambia 2006 Living Conditions Monitoring Survey) that found that over 80% of the labour force was in not formally employed.

Table 2. Socio economic characteristics, n = 88

Variable	Frequency	Percent
Fuel type		
Paraffin	1	1.1
Electricity	4	4.5
Charcoal	54	61.4
Electricity and charcoal	29	33.0
Housing status		
Low income housing	82	93.2
Medium income housing	6	6.8
Income source		
Formal	12	13.6
Informal	76	86.4
Monthly income		
Unemployed	11	12.5
Below K200	4	4.5
K200 – K500	42	47.7
Above K500	31	35.2
Spouse employment status		
Unemployed	4	4.5
Full time employment	37	42.0
Part time	12	13.6
Self employed	20	22.7
Not applicable	15	17.0
Father support		
Supported	80	90.9
Unsupported	8	9.1
Meals in a day		
1 – 3	81	92.0
4 and above	7	8.0
Source of food		
Local open market	69	78.4
Supermarket	11	12.5
Central Business District	8	9.1
Total	**88**	**100**

Only 11.4% of respondents had piped water in their dwellings, and only 10.2% were connected to a sewage system (see Table 3). Most households did not have access to solid waste collection services (58%).

Among the group with no access, 51.1% dug refuse pits around their houses, while 48.9% disposed of their waste in a stream that ran through the compound. Many households had pest and vermin, with 30.7% having a problem of cockroaches in their homes, 21.6% had both rats and cockroaches, 10.2% had cockroaches and bedbugs, 10.2% had rats only, while 27.3% had none. In the two weeks prior to our survey, 43.2% of the children had had diarrhoea (see Table 3).

Table 3. Environmental sanitation characteristics

Variable	Frequency	Percentage
Source of drinking water		
Piped in dwelling	10	11.4
Public/communal tap	78	88.6
Sanitation type (toilet)		
Flush to system	9	10.2
Ordinary pit latrine	79	89.8
Waste collection service provision		
Service present	37	42.0
No service	51	58.0
Alternative waste disposal		
Dug pit	45	51.1
Throw in nearby stream	43	48.9
Household pests and/or vermin		
Cockroaches and rats	19	21.6
Cockroaches only	27	30.7
Cockroaches and bedbugs	9	10.2
Rats only	9	10.2
None	24	27.3
Diarrhoea occurrence in children (last 2 weeks)		
Occurred	38	43.2
Did not occur	50	56.8
Overcrowding ratio		
Overcrowded	15	17.0
Adequate space	73	83.0
Total	**88**	**100**

Table 4. Knowledge levels

Variable	Frequency	Percentage (%)
Cause of Malnutrition in children		
Insufficient food	64	72.7
Bad feeding practices	15	17.0
Dirty environment, unclean water	1	1.1
Don't know	8	9.1
Water, Sanitation, Hygiene effect on nutrition		
Yes	28	31.8
No	25	28.4
Don't know	35	39.8
Total	**88**	**100**

Most parents (72.7%) attributed the cause of malnourishment to insufficient food. Others attributed it to bad feeding practices (17.0%), 1.1% dirty environment coupled with unclean water, and 9.1% did not know (see Table 4). When asked if water, sanitation, and hygiene, had any connection to nutrition in children under the age of 5, the highest percentage (39.8%) did not know, 31.8% answered in the affirmative, while 28.4% answered in the negative (see Table 4).

DISCUSSION

The study focused on malnutrition in children under the age of five years in the Chipata compound of the Lusaka District, Zambia. Using the WHO recommendations on malnutrition determination, the prevalence of underweight children was 31.8%, while the incidence of moderate to severe acute malnutrition (or wasting) was 18.2%. This study did not show that being born to a teenage mother predisposes a child to malnutrition in Chipata Compound. This was in contrast to many studies conducted in other countries that have found a significant association. Mashal et al. (16) in Afganistan (n = 2,373) and Runsewe-Aboidun and Bondi (8) in Sierra Leone (n = 406) reported that young maternal age was associated with malnourished children. However, a study by Sengupta et al. (15) with a sample size of 200 under five children randomly selected in the urban slums of Ludhiana, India, found that the mother's age did not play a major role in the child being under-weight or wasted.. Sincemore than 80% of the unmarried teenage mothers recruited into our study were living with their parents, these young mothers may have had financial support and nutrition knowledge from their family and community sufficient to mitigate malnutrition. Another reason could be the community outreach programs put in place by the Ministry of Health and executed by the Mother and Child Health unit of the Chipata First Level Hospital aimed primarily at combating malnutrition in under-fives by teaching mothers basic hygiene and nutrition.

While an educated woman is more likely to access health care, be financially empowered to provide appropriate nutrition for her children, able to exercise her reproductive rights and thereby prevent unwanted pregnancy and properly space her pregnancies, we did not find an association in this study population between the education level of the mother and child malnutrition, contrary to other studies in Zambia, Ghana, Egypt, Vietnam, and Sierra Leone (8, 16-19). This could be attributed to the family and community assistance that the mothers may have received.

We found that housing status was significantly associated with key independent variables including sanitation facility, source of drinking water, occurrence of diarrhoea, and waste collection services (see Tables 5 and 6) p-value of 0.001. Chipata compound is not a planned community and pit latrines are the most common sanitation facilities. Waste collection services are inadequate, so household waste is dumped into nearby water or refuse pits which are a breeding ground for vermin. Water contamination in the public taps is high.

Latrines and pits located close to homes predispose to food contamination and diarrheal diseases leading to malabsorption of nutrients and malnutrition.

This study showed that a very large proportion of respondents did not own their own house. It confirms a World Bank (20) report that estimated that in the poor settlements such as Chipata Compound only 35% to 40% of the residents own houses and the rest are tenants.

Table 5. p-Value summary for nutrition status by socio-demographic and socioeconomic variables

Factor	**Underweight** Number affected (%)	**Moderately to severely Malnourished** Number affected (%)
Sex of child		
Male	7(8.0))	12 (13.6)
Female	21(23.9)	4 (4.5)
p value	**0.053**	0.182
Age group of child		
6 – 23 months	22 (25.0)	16 (18.2)
24 – 59 months	5 (5.7)	0 (0.0)
p value	0.334	**0.025**
Age of mother at child birth		
13 – 19 years	4 (4.5)	3 (3.4)
20 years and above	24 (27.3)	13 (14.8)
p value	0.197	0.675
Mother's level of education		
Tertiary	1 (1.1)	2 (2.3)
Secondary	13 (14.8)	8 (9.1)
Primary	13 (14.8)	5 (5.7)
No level of education	1 (1.1)	1 (1.1)
p value	0.901	0.129
Housing status		
Low income housing	25 (28.4)	12 (13.6)
Medium income housing	3 (3.4)	4 (4.5)
High income housing	0 (0.0)	0 (0.0)
p value	0.322	**0.001**
Spouse employment status		
Full time	14 (15.9)	8 (9.1)
Part time	3 (3.4)	1 (1.1)
Self-employed	5 (5.7)	3 (3.4)
Unemployed	2 (2.3)	1 (1.1)
Not applicable	4 (4.5)	3 (3.4)
p value	0.718	0.849
Monthly income		
Unemployed	3 (3.4)	2 (2.3)
Below K200	1 (1.1)	1 (1.1)
K200 – K500	11 (12.5)	4 (4.5)
Above K500	13 (14.8)	9 (10.2)
p value	0.519	0.196
Marital status		
Single	4 (4.5)	3 (3.4)
Married	24 (27.3)	13 (14.8)
Divorced	0 (0.0)	0 (0.0)
Widowed	0 (0.0)	0 (0.0)
p value	0.571	0.681
Father support		
Yes	25 (28.4)	15 (17.0)
No	3 (3.4)	1 (1.1)
p value	0.717	0.806

Table 6. p-Value summary for Nutritional status by some environmental-related variables

Factor	Underweight No. (%)	Moderately to Severely Malnourished No. (%)
Source of water		
Piped in dwelling	1 (1.1)	2 (2.3)
Public tap	27 (30.7)	14 (15.9)
p value	0.116	0.874
Waste collection service		
Yes	14 (15.9)	7 (8.0)
No	14 (15.9)	9 (10.2)
p value	0.302	0.879
Alternative disposal option		
Dug pit	10 (11.4)	8 (9.1)
Nearby stream	7 (8.0)	3 (3.4)
Not applicable	11 (12.5)	5 (5.7)
p value	0.720	0.294
Sanitary type		
Flush to sewerage system	2 (2.3)	1 (1.1)
Ordinary pit latrine	26 (29.5)	15 (17.0)
p value	0.514	0.562
Food source		
Local street vendor	23 (26.1)	10 (11.4)
Local supermarket	2 (2.3)	3 (3.4)
Central Business District	3 (3.4)	3 (3.4)
p value	0.567	0.197
Diarrhoea occurrence in last 2 weeks		
Yes	13 (14.8)	8 (9.1)
No	15 (17.0)	8 (9.1)
p value	0.674	0.543
Number of inhabitants		
Between 1 and 5	19 (21.6)	8 (9.1)
Between 6 and 10	9 (10.2)	8 (9.1)
Above 10	0 (0.0)	0 (0.0)
p value	0.217	**0.009**

Note:

1. The total number of children found with the two types of malnutrition under investigation was 44; in columns 2 and 3 the numbers of those malnourished are shown, with the representative percentage indicated in parentheses.
2. The tables 5 and 6 are summaries of cross tabulations between the dependent variable *nutrition status* against independent variables. *p*-values are indicated below each cross tabulation. These were generated by the statistical package SPSS.

Housing status was significantly associated with variables such as sanitation, source of drinking water, and the number of household members. Furthermore, housing status and number of household members were highly significant risk factors for malnutrition. This implied that children living in low cost houses were at a very high risk of being malnourished. In the study population, women with limited education and income had limited housing options. Therefore, they settled in infrastructure that was inadequate, exposing them to environmental health hazards such as indoor air pollution, poor sanitation, and contaminated underground water. When disease such as diarrhea results from these hazards, it brings about poor nutrition and inadequate physical activity in both the mother and under- five child. Malnourished children are less able to participate fully at school. Stunted women are less productive and more likely to give birth to low-birth-weight babies. A low-birth-weight infant is more likely to be 'stunted' (low height-for-age) by the age of 5 years. Such a child, without adequate food, health and care, will become a 'stunted' adolescent and later, a 'stunted' adult, perpetuating the cycle of malnutrition from generation to generation.

Figure 1 depicts this cycle of environmental health disparities affecting the under-five-years children in the study population. These are the points at which various interventions can be targeted. Some key interventions include introduction of school re-entry programs for young girls who become pregnant and health promotion focusing on nutrition for the mothers and their under five children.

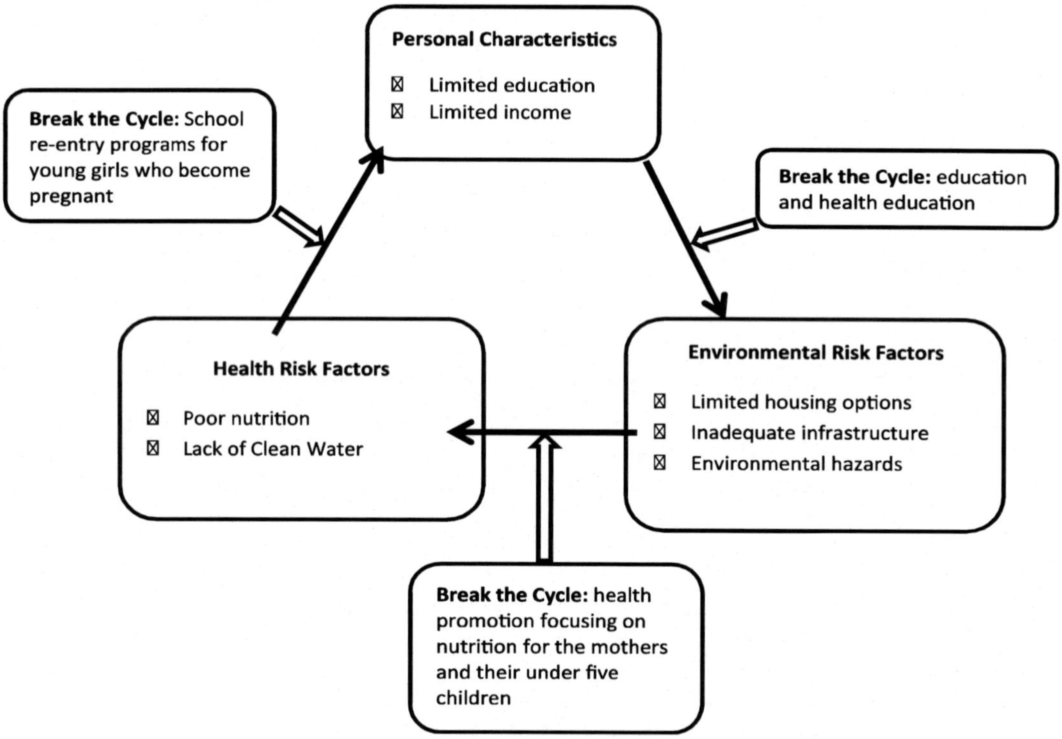

Figure 1. Cycle of environmental health disparities in the study population.

Implementing programs to improve maternal education and earning power would empower them to choose healthier housing options and give them knowledge to prepare more nutritious meals for their families, thereby reducing exposure to environmental hazards and malnutrition. Consequently, both the mother and the child will be more likely to be in good health. The mother will then be able to engage in economically helpful activities while the child will have a higher likelihood of normal physical and mental development and this way breake the cycle of disadvantage and disability.

ACKNOWLEDGMENTS

Special thanks to Mrs. Munyinda for her guidance and support throughout this project. Thanks also to the "Break the Cycle" team for encouraging my participation in this project.

REFERENCES

[1] World Health Organization. Safer water, better health: Costs, benefits and sustainability of interventions to protect and promote health, 2008. URL: http://www.who.int.

[2] Simiyu S. Water risk factors pre-disposing the under five children to diarrhoeal morbidity in Mandera district, Kenya. East Afr J Public Health 2010;7:353-360.

[3] UNICEF. The state of the world's children. New York: UNICEF, 2006.

[4] World Health Organization. Essential nutrition actions: Improving maternal, newborn, infant and young child health and nutrition, 2013. URL: http://www.ncbi.nlm.nih.gov/books/NBK258736.

[5] Katepa-Bwalya M. Feeding practices and nutritional status of infants and young children in Mazabuka and Kafue districts of Zambia. Lusaka: University of Zambia, 2008.

[6] Burgess A, Danga L. Under nutrition in adults and children: causes, consequences and what we can do. Sudan Med Bull 2008;1:1:8-13.

[7] Lawn JE, Simon C, Jelka Z. 4 Million neonatal deaths: When? Where? Why? Lancet 2005;365;9462:347.

[8] Tamramat I, Runsewe-Abiodun and Bondi SF. Teenage pregnancy and implications on child survival amongst mothers attending a clinic in the East-End. Open J Pediatrics 2013;3:294-9.

[9] Nyaruhucha CNM, Msuya JM, Mamiro PS, Kerengi AJ. Nutritional status and feeding practices of under-five children in Simanjiro District, Tanzania. Tanzan Health Res Bull 2006;8:162-7.

[10] TRCH. Tanzania reproductive and child health survey 1999. Calverton, MD: Bureau Statistics, Macro International, 2000.

[11] USAID. Nutrition of infants and young children in Tanzania, 1997. Washington, DC: African Nutrition Chartbooks, USAID, 1998.

[12] Beaglehole R, Bonita R. Public health cross road achievement and prospects. London: Cambridge University Press, 1997.

[13] Vorster HH and Hautvast J. A Global perspective on food and nutrition. In: Gibney MJ, Vorster HH, Kok FJ, eds. The Nutrition Society Textbook Series. Introduction to human nutrition. Osdney Mead, Oxford: Blackwell Science, 2002:5-6.

[14] Mashal T, Takano T, Nakamura K, Kizuki M, Hemat S, Watanabe M, et al. Factors associated with the health and nutritional status of children under 5 years of age in Afghanistan: Family behaviour related to women and past experience of war-related hardships. BMC Public Health 2008;8:301.

[15] Sengupta P, Philip, N, Benjamin AI. Epidemiological correlates of under-nutrition in under-5 years children in an urban slum of Ludhiana. Health Populat Perspect Issues 2010;33(1):1.

[16] Nzala SH, Siziya S, Babaniyi O, Songolo P, Muula A, Rudatsikira E. Demographic, cultural and environmental factors associated with frequency and severity of malnutrition among Zambia children less than five years of age. J Public Health Epidemiol 2011;3(8):362-70.

[17] Appoh LY, Krekling S. Maternal nutritional knowledge and child nutritional status in the Volta region of Ghana. Matern Child Nutr 2005;1:100-10.

[18] Zottarelli LK, Sunil TS, Rajaram S. Influence of parental and socioeconomic factors on stunting in children under 5 years in Egypt. East Mediterr Health J 2007;13:1330-42.

[19] Hien NN, Kam S. Nutritional status and the characteristics related to malnutrition in children under five years of age in Nghean, Vietnam. J Prev Med Public Health 2008;41: 232-40.

[20] Mulenga CL. Understanding slums: case studies for the global report 2003. Lusaka: Institute Economic Social Research, University of Zambia, 2003.

[21] UN-HABITAT. Rental housing: An essential option for the urban poor in developing countries. UN-HABITAT 2003. URL: http://www.unhabitat.org/books/rental-housing-an-essential-option-for-the-urban-poor-in-developing-countries.

In: Environmental Health Disparities
Editors: I Leslie Rubin and Joav Merrick

ISBN: 978-1-63484-211-2

Chapter 3

RACIAL CONCENTRATION AND ACCESS TO HEALTH CARE IN GEORGIA

Shruthi Satyamurthy*, DDS, MBA/MHA, and Daniel Montanera, PhD
Institute of Health Administration,
J Mack Robinson College of Business,
Georgia State University,
Atlanta, Georgia, US

The legacy of racial segregation in the Southeast United States has resulted in substantial variation in neighborhood racial concentration in Georgia. This variation among neighborhoods has been implicated as a contributing factor in higher risk of chronic diseases, increased infant mortality rate, and low birthweight among minorities. This article attempts to estimate the effects of this neighborhood-level racial concentration on individuals' access to health care, while controlling for individual-level characteristics. It does so by linking individual-level data from an independently conducted survey with neighborhood-level characteristics through respondents' zip codes. Findings reveal a significant negative correlation between the concentrations of black residents in an individual's neighborhood both with that individual's visits to a health care facility and with satisfaction with access to health care, even after controlling for individual characteristics. This suggests the presence of access barriers that disproportionately affect black neighborhoods. The implication is, rather than attempt access expansions at low-income or unemployed individuals, not-for-profit organizations and policymakers should pursue neighborhood- or community-level projects to most effectively overcome health care access disparities.

* Correspondence: Shruthi Satyamurthy, Institute of Health Administration, Robinson College of Business, 35 Broad Street NW, Suite 805, PO Box 3988, Atlanta, GA 30302-3988, United States. E-mail: shru.sam13@gmail.com.

INTRODUCTION

Despite the implementation of the Affordable Care Act (ACA), disparities in access to health care still exist today in the United States. Many Americans remain uninsured and dissatisfied with their personal access to healthcare. There are many possible reasons for this disparity in access, including socio-economic, environmental, behavioral, biological, and genetic factors. One of the most significant contributors, however, is Racial Residential Segregation (RRS). RRS today is the concentration of personal residence, based on race, into certain geographic areas (1). In the past, this included legally restricted residence in some areas of the country. The possible mechanisms through which RRS could affect health include racial bias in medical care, low access to health insurance, and poor access to health care facilities. The Affordable Care Act attempts to expand access to care primarily at the individual-level, though efforts like the expansion of Medicaid. In targeting the individual, however, it does not address neighborhood-level problems like RRS, and could therefore allow racial disparities in access to care to persist.

Segregation has been prevalent in Georgia since 1900, when majority of the black community moved into urban areas (2). There were also several segregation laws implemented in the past. A majority of Southeast American states enforced segregation through "Jim Crow" laws (3-6), examples of which include prohibition of interracial marriages and racial segregation of public schools (7). These laws created de jure segregation by race, and further regulated social, economic, and political relationships between whites and African-Americans (8, 9). Segregation was not only common in the southern United States, but also present in a de facto sense in the north (10). Blacks could not buy houses in the same neighborhoods as whites and economic and educational opportunities for black Americans were greatly restricted (11). This illustrates the institutional foundation for how RRS arose in the United States and how it could persist even after the Jim Crow laws were repealed (12).

Evidence of racial disparities in access to health care is well established in the United States. Majority black communities have experienced discrimination in relatively depressed housing policies, bank loans, labor markets, and real estate transactions (13). Furthermore, as late as 1995, primarily black communities have suffered more from environmental degradation than primarily white ones (14), Residents face disparities in quality of education, educational attainment, employment opportunities, income and health insurance status; all of which contribute to disparities in access to health care (15). Blacks are more likely than whites to be uninsured or covered by Medicaid (16). The result is that blacks utilize health services at lower rates than whites (15, 17, 18), even when comparing individuals with similar health needs (19). Blacks living in more segregated areas have less comprehensive health insurance coverage compared to blacks living in less segregated areas (20). Low private health insurance coverage, and the resulting poor reimbursement rates, could create difficulties for those health care facilities and providers serving black communities. Poor access to care has, in turn, contributed to increased incidences of asthma and cardio-vascular disease (17). The pattern is also observable in infant health, where "there were 1.12 excess infant deaths per thousand live births among black infants due to living in a segregated city compared with a non-segregated city" (21). Taken together, the evidence suggests that segregation is a potentially important variable in explaining persistent racial disparities in access to health care.

The fact that a neighborhood is partly defined by its individual residents creates challenges in estimating the impact of neighborhood-level racial concentration on access to health care. Due to the correlations between race, education level, income, unemployment, health insurance, and health outcomes described above, there are bound to be correlations between the racial concentration of a neighborhood and the socio-economic characteristics of the residents. In regressions of access measures on neighborhood characteristics, these confounding factors create problems in interpreting coefficients as causal effects. For this reason, in estimating the marginal impact of RRS on access to health care, it is important to separate the individual- and neighborhood-level characteristics as explanatory variables.

OUR STUDY

This study attempts to quantify the effect of racial concentration, independently of individual characteristics, on access to health care. It does so by first conducting an independent survey of individual socioeconomic characteristics, health care utilization, and perceptions of access to health care. Next, individuals are linked to neighborhood-level characteristics through the individual's stated zip code in the survey. The study then proceeds with ordinary least-squares regression to identify the individual- and neighborhood-level variables most predictive of health care utilization and satisfaction with access to care. Results show that, even when controlling for individual characteristics, the concentration of black residents in a neighborhood is strongly negatively correlated with both health care utilization and perceived access to care. This suggests that community-level interventions designed to overcome barriers to access may prove more successful than those solely targeting individuals.

Separating individual- and neighborhood-level contributors to poor health care access requires data with detailed individual characteristics linked to the characteristics of that individual's neighborhood. A questionnaire was prepared for both online and written surveys of respondents' individual characteristics. The questionnaire was divided into two sections: demographic information and access to health care. The demographic section (see Table 1) requests that respondents report age, gender, ethnicity, education, employment status, household income, dependents, and zip code. The section concerning access to care (see Table 2) contains questions regarding respondents' health insurance status, type of health insurance plan, typical number of visits to a health care facility per year, level of satisfaction with personal access to health care, typical mode of transportation to health care facilities, and the number of facilities to which the respondent could travel within a given timeframe. The online version of the questionnaire was conducted through Qualtrics survey (22) and distributed by word of mouth and social media (primarily Facebook). Written surveys were distributed in person by the authors in public venues in the City of Atlanta, primarily at Lenox Square. The survey garnered 75 total responses, of which 13 were written and 62 online. Accounting for incomplete surveys or missing answers to key variables left a total of 69 responses as observations in the analysis.

Variables placing respondents in categories (age, education, household income, distance to closest health care facility, and number of visits to a health care facility) assigned a value of 0 to the lowest category (Option “A” in the survey) and increased by 1 for each subsequent category. A respondent was categorized as “other race” if any of “Native American or American Indian, Asian, Mixed, or Other” was indicated on the questionnaire. The respondent’s employment status variable was set equal to zero if unemployed, one if employed part-time, and two if employed full-time.

Table 1. Demographic Questionnaire

1. What is your age? a. 18-24 years old b. 25-34 years old c. 35-44 years old d. 45-54 years old e. 55-64 years old f. 65-74 years old 2. What is your gender? a. Female b. Male 3. Which best describes your ethnicity? a. White b. Hispanic or Latino c. Black or African American d. Native American or American Indian e. Asian f. Mixed g. Other 4. What is the highest level of schooling completed or degree achieved? a. Less than high school degree b. High school degree or equivalent c. Associate degree d. Bachelor degree e. Graduate degree 5. What is your marital status? a. Married b. Widowed c. Divorced d. Separated e. Never married 6. Do you have any dependents (a person relying on you for their daily needs)? a. Yes b. No	7. A. What is the number of dependents? a. 1 b. 2 c. 3 or more B. Is a parent one of your dependent (s)? C. Is a spouse one of your dependent(s)? D. Is a child one of your dependent(s)? a. Yes b. No 8. What is your total household income? a. Less than $10,000 b. $10,000 to $20,999 c. $30,000 to $59,999 d. $60,000 to $89,999 e. $90,000 to $149,999 f. More than $150,000 9. Which of the following best describes your current employment status? a. Employed for wages Full- Time b. Employed for wages Part- Time c. Self-employed Full- Time d. Self- employed Part-Time e. Not employed 10. Are you actively seeking another job? a. Yes b. No 11. What is your five digit Zip code of your primary residence? (For Example: 576, Pleasant View Parade, Yonkers, Georgia– 35163). Please provide the Zip code in the space provided. -- --

Table 2. Access Questionnaire

1. What is the source of your health insurance?

a. Medicaid
b. Medicare
c. Dual eligible (Medicaid and Medicare)
d. Employer based (Through your work place)
e. Federal health insurance exchange (Healthcare.gov)
f. No insurance

2. Which of the following best describes your health insurance plan?

a. HMO- Health maintenance organization
b. PPO- Preferred Provider Organization
c. POS- Point of service
d. Open network (No restriction on provider)
e. Military
f. No health insurance
g. Not sure
h. Other: ____________________________

3. Approximately how far (distance in miles) is the closest health care facility (Hospitals, physician office, clinics) from your home?

a. 0-2
b. 3-5
c. 6-15
d. 16- 25
e. 26-35
f. More than 35
g. Not sure

4.
A. How many health care facilities could you get to in 15 minutes?
B. How many health care facilities could you get to in half an hour?
C. How many health care facilities could you get to in one hour?

a. 0
b. 1
c. 2
d. 3-5
e. 5 or more

5. How many times per year do you visit a health care facility for treatment?

a. Less than 1
b. 1 – 3
c. 4 – 6
d. 7 – 9
e. 9 – 11
f. 12 or more

6. What is your main mode of transportation for reaching your health care facility?

a. Car
b. A ride/lift in someone else's car
c. Bus
d. MARTA
e. Taxi
f. By Walk
g. Other

7. Which of the following best describes your personal access to healthcare?

a. Excellent
b. Very Good
c. Good
d. Poor

A similar practice was followed for the payer of the respondent's health insurance: zero if uninsured, 1 if the payer is public (Medicare/Medicaid or dual eligible), and 2 if the payer is private through either a health insurance exchange or the workplace. Two dummy variables were created for respondents' typical modes of transportation when visiting health care facilities, one each for automobile and public transit. Satisfaction with access to health care was set equal to zero if the respondent indicated "poor" in the survey, and increases by one with each category up to 4, indicating "excellent." Both satisfaction with access to care and the number of visits to a health care facility are used in this article as measures of patient access to health care.

Neighborhood characteristics, such as racial concentration and male/female population by zip code, were obtained from City-Data, administered by Advameg, Inc. It is a social networking and information website, presenting data and information pertaining to US cities. In general, their database contains demographic data, real estate, employment status, crime history, air pollution, weather patterns, food environment statistics, agriculture, religion, incidents of natural calamity and government finances expenditure (23). Further neighborhood characteristics, such as average household income and population by zip code, was obtained from ZipAtlas. This database also provides information on unemployment rates, industry statistics, household and personal income reports, and property value assessment, housing unit occupancy and vacancy breakdown and mortgage and rent analysis (24). Finally, data on the proximity of health care facilities to various zip codes was obtained through the Dartmouth Atlas of Healthcare. It documents variations in how medical resources are distributed and used in the United States. It uses Medicare data to provide information and analysis about national, regional, local markets as well as individual hospitals and their affiliated physicians (25).

This study uses an index to capture the degree of racial concentration in a neighborhood. It does this in order to separate the pure segregation effect (resulting from the racial homogeneity of the neighborhood) from the race-specific concentration (the share of neighborhood residents of a particular race). The variable "*concindex*" (see Table 3) is a version of the Herfindahl-Hirschman Index (HHI), except using each ethnicity's share of the total population instead of each firm's market share. Therefore, *concindex* reaches a maximum value of 1 for those neighborhoods that are ethnically homogenous (for any of black, white, or other ethnicity), and a minimum value of 1/3 in the potential case where neighborhood residents are evenly distributed among the three ethnicities. The percentage of neighborhood residents who are black is included as a separate variable "*Zpercblack*" in order to capture how different ethnicities are affected by racial concentration.

FINDINGS

The summary statistics characterizing survey respondents are presented in Tables 3 and 4. They show that the typical survey respondent is in the age range of 35 to 44 years.

Table 3. Summary Statistics of Sample Individual and Neighborhood Characteristics

Variable	Mean	Std. deviation	Min	Max
Male	0.26	0.44	0	1
Black	0.47	0.50	0	1
Other Race	0.18	0.39	0	1
Zincome	48773.25	16288.73	19k	95k
Zpercblack	0.37	0.31	0.026	0.97
Concindex	0.63	0.14	0.36	0.94
Zhospfive	2.16	2.31	0	8
Zhospten	5.41	3.38	0	11

Table 4. Distribution and Median of Age, Income, Payer and Employment variables

Variable	Responses	Distribution (in %)	Median
Age (years)	0: 18- 24 1: 25-34 2: 35-44 3: 45-54 4: 55-64 5: 65-74	23.19 36.23 15.94 15.94 7.25 1.45	25-34 years
Income	0: less than 10,000 1: 10,000- 20,999 2: 30,000- 59,999 3: 60,000- 89,999 4: 90,000- 149999 5: more than 150,000	7.35 13.24 38.24 16.18 17.65 7.35	30,000- 60,000
Employed	0: Not employed 1: Employed/self employed- Part time 2: Employed/self employed: Full time	13.04 18.84 68.12	Employed Full time
Payer	0: No insurance 1: Medicare, Medicaid, dual eligible 2: Employer based, Federal health insurance	15.94 4.35 79.71	Employer-based, Federal health insurance

The respondents are heavily skewed towards female (74%), which is a caveat as this does not accurately represent the distribution of sexes in Georgia. At 48%, blacks are significantly over-represented among respondents when compared to the Georgia population (30%). There were no Hispanic respondents.

Typical household income of respondents is between $30,000 and $60,000, consistent with mean income of $48,773 at the zip code level. Respondents' stated neighborhoods varied substantially, with no more than four respondents indicating the same zip code. The variable *Zpercblack* from Table 3 has a standard deviation roughly equal to its mean, and the range of *concindex* covers nearly all possible values of the index. Therefore, this sample of respondents contains sufficient variation to attempt to uncover the effect of racial concentration on access to health care.

Using OLS regression, this article estimates the following empirical model:

$$y_{ij} = a + X_i\beta + Z_{ij}\gamma + \varepsilon_i \qquad (1)$$

where y_{ij} is either respondent *i*'s personal satisfaction with their access to health care or the number of visits that respondent *i* makes to a health care facility in a typical year. The vector

X_i contains individual-level demographic variables including dummies for age, male, and race (one each for black and other).

Also included are variables indicating categories for total household income, marital status, and the type of payer behind the respondent's health insurance (uninsured, public, or private). The vector Z_{ij} contains the neighborhood-level characteristics linked to respondent *i*'s stated zip code of residence *j* in the questionnaire. These variables include the concentration index (*concindex*), percentage of residents who are black (*Zpercblack*), mean household income, and number of hospitals within five- and ten-mile distances of the zip code.

Table 5 shows the results of estimating Equation (1) using personal satisfaction with access to health care as the dependent variable. The most important individual-level characteristics affecting this measure of access are the payer sponsoring the respondent's health insurance (significant at the 5% level) and the respondent's income (borderline significant at the 5% level). Not surprisingly, both coefficients are positive, which indicates that greater income and having publicly- or privately-sponsored health insurance is likely to increase a respondent's personal satisfaction with their access to health care. The respondent's race is an insignificant determinant of access to care while the concentration of blacks in the respondent's neighborhood is statistically significant at the 10% level. The estimated coefficient of -1.30 reveals the prediction that, all else being equal, the resident of an entirely black neighborhood would report more than one full category lower satisfaction with access to health care, compared to a resident of an entirely non-black neighborhood. The estimates also show that this correlation exists independently of the surveyed characteristics of the respondent, and is not the result of racial segregation alone, as shown by the insignificant coefficient on the concentration index variable. Therefore, racial concentration has an asymmetrically negative effect on the satisfaction with access to health care of the residents of largely black neighborhoods.

There is an interesting relationship between the number of hospitals within five and ten miles of the respondent's neighborhood and the respondent's satisfaction with access to health care. For each hospital within a five-mile radius. Table 5 shows a small negative correlation with the respondent's satisfaction, significant at the 10% level. Conversely, each hospital within a ten-mile radius has a small positive correlation with satisfaction, significant at the 5% level. This indicates that respondents' access to health care improves when hospitals are close, but not too close. One possible explanation for this involves the profile of neighborhood in which hospitals typically locate.

A negative correlation would be expected if hospitals tend to locate in undesirable residential areas, and if the residents of these areas typically have poor access to care for a variety of reasons. Therefore, the negative effect of number of hospitals within five miles is likely due to these confounding factors, with hospital proximity in general having a positive marginal effect on patient satisfaction overall.

The second proxy for access to health care is examined in Table 6. The number of visits the respondent makes to a health care facility in a typical year is used as the dependent variable in Equation (1). For this access measure, none of the individual characteristics is a significant determinant. Regarding neighborhood-level characteristics, the coefficient of mean zip code income is negative and significant at the 5% level, and implies a neighborhood-level income elasticity of -1.73.

Table 5. Effects of Individual- and Neighborhood-Level Characteristics on Satisfaction with Access to Health Care

Satisfaction	**Coefficient**	**Std. Error**
Black	0.28	0.34
Age	-0.09	0.12
Otherrace	-0.32	0.33
Income	0.20*	0.10
Employed	0.03	0.21
Payer	0.72**	0.19
Zincome	-7.9e	0.0012
Zpercblack	-1.30*	0.73
Concindex	1.63	1.11
Zhospfive	-0.16*	0.092
Zhospten	0.14**	0.064

R Squared: 0.4212.
Number of observations: 62.
"*" indicates significance at the 10% level.
"**" indicates significance at the 5% level.

Table 6. Effects of Individual- and Neighborhood-Level Characteristics on Visits per Year to a Healthcare Facility

Visits per year	**Coefficient**	**Std. Error**
Black	0.35	0.37
Age	0.80	0.14
Otherrace	0.69*	0.40
Income	0.06	0.12
Employed	-0.04	0.24
Payer	0.20	0.21
Zincome	-0.00039**	0.000014
Zpercblack	-1.83**	0.78
Concindex	0.53	1.21
Zhospfive	-0.15	0.10
Zhospten	-0.0037	0.073

R Squared: 0.2234.
Number of Observations: 66.
*" indicates significance at the 10% level.
"**" indicates significance at the 5% level.

The relationship between the number of visits and the concentration of black residents in the neighborhood is also negative and significant at the 5% level, implying an elasticity of -0.62. A fifty percentage-point increase in the share of neighborhood residents who are black is associated with one fewer visit to a health care facility in a typical year per neighborhood resident. Note that this is the same qualitative effect that was found when using patient satisfaction as the dependent variable. Together, the estimated effects of the concentration measures on both patient satisfaction and health care visits reveal compelling evidence that the residents of predominantly black neighborhoods suffer poorer access to health care due to residential racial segregation.

DISCUSSION

Even in the United States today, there exist disparities across races in access to and utilization of quality health care, contributing to adverse outcomes in infant mortality, low birthweight, morbidity, and mortality in vulnerable populations. This study investigates the impact of Racial Residential Segregation (RRS) on individual access to health care in Georgia. Such investigation is important given the legacy of enforced racial segregation and the existing evidence of poorer health outcomes in largely black communities. Accounting for the endogenous nature of individual location decisions requires separating the individual- and neighborhood-level characteristics in order to determine the pure marginal effect of neighborhood racial concentration on access measures. The results show that, even controlling for relevant individual characteristics, the concentration of black residents in a neighborhood is one of the most important predictors of access to health care among that neighborhood's residents. This holds where access in measured in both personal satisfaction and in the number of visits to a health care facility in a typical year. This implies that Racial Residential Segregation, in addition to other social problems, is a public and environmental health problem where access to care in largely black neighborhoods suffers as a result.

The exact mechanism through which segregation might affect access to care is not clear. Presuming that the individual characteristics included in this analysis reasonably proxy for demand-side factors, then the most likely explanation may lie with the supply side of the health services market. For a variety of social, political, and economic reasons, health insurers and providers may have lacked the incentive to locate, engage with, or reach out to neighborhoods with high concentrations of black residents. Neglecting these neighborhoods may be a form of indirect risk selection if suppliers perceive these residents to be high-risk or unprofitable patients.

These findings have important implications for policymakers and not-for-profit organizations concerned with community health and access to care. The primary goal of the Affordable Care Act is the expansion of access to health care, and largely does so by conditioning Medicaid coverage and premium subsidies on individual or household income. The analysis conducted here indicates that neighborhood racial concentration is a more important, consistent, and significant predictor of access to care than any of the collected individual factors. This suggests that the country's current national health strategy may fail to unlock the tremendous potential to expand access to health care through neighborhood or community projects. Based on findings above, these projects are an effective way to expand access to health care, and thus improve the limited healthcare services identified as a compounding risk factor in Figure 1.

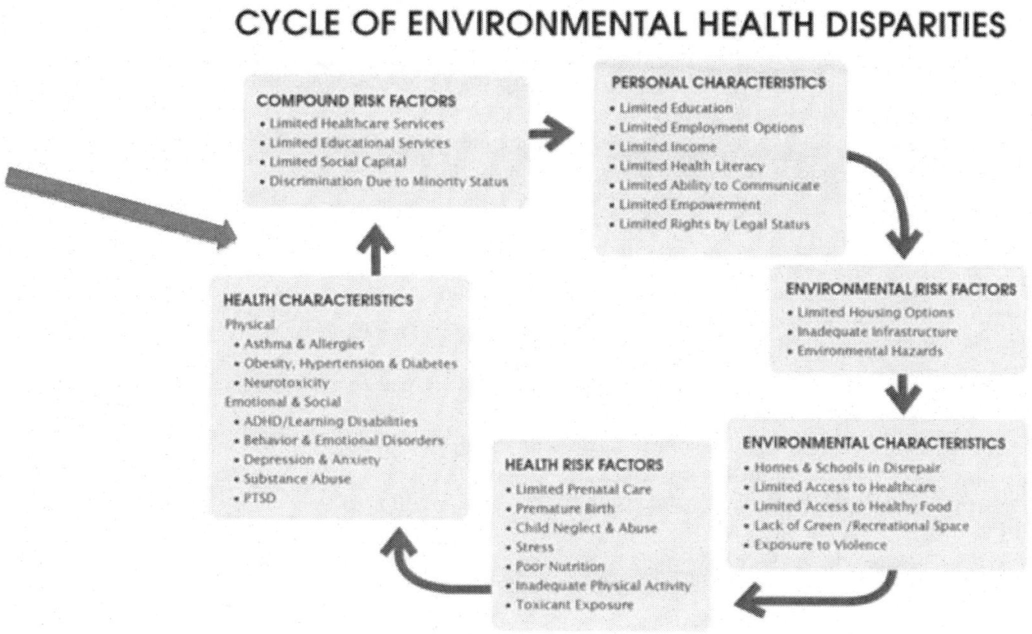

Figure 1. The Cycle of Environmental Health Disparities.

In this way, initiatives like improved housing conditions; inter-community health, employment, education centers; and adequate public transit to facilitate the use of health care facilities can be effective in breaking the cycle of environmental health disparities. There are a few limitations in this study. First, despite controlling for several important individual characteristics, there may remain unobserved variables correlated with both individual access to health care and individuals' neighborhood of residence. While this somewhat complicates the interpretation of the estimated relationships as causal, the individual variables included in the study (age, race, income, employment, and insurance sponsor) are likely to capture a great deal of the individual-level effects on place of residence.

Second, given the research topic and the personal nature of access to health care, the survey may have attracted a sample of respondents who are particularly sensitive to the subject. This source of bias is likely to be less important in the estimated effects of neighborhood characteristics, however, since these were not directly solicited in the questionnaire, but were linked to the respondent's stated zip code. This reduces the likelihood that individuals' perceptions surrounding access to care in their neighborhoods might distort the estimated effects.

Finally, the survey obtained a small sample of respondents with several characteristics that do not match the general population of Georgia. There may also be some selection bias among respondents given the media through which the survey was conducted. For example, vulnerable sub-populations in Georgia may lack the internet access necessary to complete an online survey distributed through social media. Despite these limitations, the relationships uncovered in this article strongly suggest that residential racial segregation is an important and often overlooked factor in community and environmental health of vulnerable populations, and worthy of further investigation.

REFERENCES

[1] Williams RD, Collins C. Racial residential segregation: a fundamental cause of racial disparities in health. Public Health Rep 2001;116(5):404-16.

[2] Smelser NJ, Wilson WJ, Mitchell F, eds. America becoming: Racial trends and their consequences. Volume I. Washington, DC: National Academy Press, 2001.

[3] Jim Crow Laws. URL: http://www.nps.gov/malu/learn/education/jim_crow_laws.htm.

[4] Seitles M. The perpetuation of residential racial segregation in America: Historical discrimination, modern forms of exclusion, and inclusionary remedies. J Land Use Environ Law 1996. URL: http://archive.law.fsu.edu/journals/landuse/Vol141/seit.htm.

[5] Kosman J. Toward an inclusionary jurisprudence: A reconceptualization of zoning. Catholic Univ Law Rev 1993;43:59-108.

[6] Oh R. Interracial marriage in the shadows of Jim Crow. Racial segregation as a system of racial and gender subordination. UC Davis Law Rev 2005;39:1321-52.

[7] Massey DS, Denton NA. American apartheid: Segregation and the making of the underclass. Cambridge, MA: Harvard University Press, 1993.

[8] Tischauser LV. Jim Crow laws. Santa Barbara, CA: ABC-CLIO, 2012.

[9] Kousser JM. Jim Crow laws. In: Dictionary of American History, 3rd ed. New York: Charles Scribner's Sons, 2003:479-80.

[10] Douglas DM. Jim Crow moves morth: The battle over northern school desegregation, 1865- 1954. New York: Cambridge University Press, 2005.

[11] Racial segregation in the American South: Jim Crow laws. In: Rudd K, Hanes R, Hermsen S, eds. Prejudice in the Modern World Reference Library Detroit, MI: Gale Global Issues, 2007;2:333-57.

[12] De Leeuw MB, Whyte MK, Ho D, Meza C, Karteron A. Residential segregation and housing discrimination in the United States: Violations of the International Convention on the Elimination of All Forms of Racial Discrimination. URL: http://www. ushrnetwork. org/files/ushrn/images/ linkfiles/CERD/17_Housing%20Discrimination. pdf(2007).

[13] Massey DS, Denton NA. The dimensions of residential segregation. Soc Forces 1988;67(2):281-315.

[14] Collins C, Williams DR. Examining the black-white adult mortality disparity: The role of residential segregation. Heart Disease 1995;213:1-45.

[15] Landrine H, Corral I. Separate and unequal: Residential segregation and Black health disparities. Ethnicity Dis 2009;19:179-84.

[16] DeNavas-Walt C, Proctor BD, Smith JC. US Census Bureau. Income, poverty, and health insurance coverage in the United States, 2009. Washington, DC: US Government Printing Office, 2010.

[17] Gaskin DJ, Dinwiddie GY, Chan KS, McCleary R. Residential segregation and disparities in health care services utilization. Med Care Res Rev 2012;69(2):158-75.

[18] US Department of Health and Human Services, Agency for Healthcare Research and Quality. National Healthcare Disparities Report, 2007. Rockville, MD: Agency for Healthcare Research and Quality, 2008.

[19] Andersen RM. Revisiting the behavioral model and access to medical care: Does it matter? J Health Soc Behav 1995;36(1):1–10.

[20] Anderson KF, Fullerton AS, Kronenfeld JJ. Racial residential segregation and access to health-care coverage: A multilevel analysis. Bingley, UK: Emerald Group Publishing, 2012.

[21] Hearst MO, Oakes JM, Johnson PJ. The effect of racial residential segregation on Black infant mortality. Am J Epidemiology 2008;168(11):1247-54.

[22] Qualtrics software. Qualtrics, Provo, UT. Version March 2015; Copyright 2015 URL: http://www.gsu.qualtrics.com.

[23] Georgia Bigger Cities [Internet] 2012 March. URL: http://www.city-data.com/city/Atlanta-Georgia.html.

[24] Zip Codes with the Highest Median Household Income in Georgia [Internet] 2013. URL: http://zipatlas.com/us/ga/zip-code-comparison/median-household-income.htm.

[25] Data by hospital. The Dartmouth Atlas of Healthcare. [Internet] 2010. URL http://www. dartmouthatlas.org/data/hospital/?zip=30096&distance=10 9.

In: Environmental Health Disparities
Editors: I Leslie Rubin and Joav Merrick

ISBN: 978-1-63484-211-2

Chapter 4

LIVING NEAR NUCLEAR POWER PLANTS

Christina Sauer*, BA, Julie Strominger, MS, and Pamela Maxson, PhD
School of Natural Resources and the Environment,
University of Michigan, Ann Arbor, Michigan, US

In this chapter, we assess racial and socioeconomic (SES) disparities in the population living near an active nuclear power plant across the Eastern United States. Unlike similar prior studies of environmental justice aspects in nuclear power plant siting using data at the census-tract level, we look at racial and SES disparities among children and families living near nuclear power plants at a finer spatial scale, the block-group level, in the Eastern United States. This study seeks to elucidate the environmental justice implications of living near a nuclear power plant in the Eastern United States.

INTRODUCTION

Until 1994, environmental laws and health protection standards did not protect racial minority and low socio-economic status (SES) communities (1). By 1994, the term "environmental justice" was legally instituted through Presidential Executive Order 12898. Environmental justice is "the fair treatment and meaningful involvement of all people regardless of race, color, national origin or income with respect to the development, implementation, and enforcement of environmental laws, regulations, and policies" (2).

Underprivileged populations are at an increased risk of adverse health outcomes, such as asthma, and disproportionately exposed to environmental stressors like ozone and particulate matter < 2.5μm in aerodynamic matter (3). Little research has focused on environmental justice regarding exposure to radiation emitted from nuclear power plants.

Nearly 40% of the United States population lives within 50 miles of a nuclear facility (4). All current operating nuclear plants, with the exception of the Vogtle nuclear reactors in Waynesboro, Georgia, were built prior to Executive Order 12898 without consideration for

* Correspondence: Christina Sauer, 2751 German Ridge Road Northeast, Corydon, IN 47112, United States. E-mail: cmsauer@umich.edu; sauer.christina.m@gmail.com.

racial and socioeconomic disparities in the construction region. The California Waste Management Board purposefully identified ideal sites for "undesirable land uses" as conservative rural populations with low incomes and higher education rates with the "least potential of generating public opposition" (5). Numerous studies have documented the environmental injustices surrounding uranium mining and waste disposal facilities and occupational hazards for nuclear plant workers (6) However, only two studies have evaluated environmental injustices in the populations residing near nuclear power plants in the eastern United States (4, 6).

Previous research has examined the relationship between adverse health outcomes such as leukemia and distance to a nuclear facility as a proxy for exposure to low levels of ionizing radiation emitted from a facility (7). Researchers in Germany, France, and the United Kingdom found that children residing within 5 kilometers (approximately 3 miles) of a nuclear power plant were at an increased risk of developing cancer (7, 8).

In the United States, the National Cancer Institute found that children living roughly within 30 miles of a nuclear power plant are exposed to low-level doses of radiation (9). The 2006 publication of the BEIR VII elicited questions into the current radiation protection standards as it indicated that no level of radiation is safe for children (10). All acceptable levels of regulated radiation emissions from nuclear power plants are based on a protection standard, 'Reference Man.' Reference Man was established in 1975 by the International Commission on Radiological Protection that defined the average individual as a Caucasian male between the ages of 20 and 30 years old, weighing 70 kg (154 pounds) and 170 cm (5 feet 7 inches) tall. This protection standard fails miserably to include children with their body weight, height, metabolism and growing organs and organ systems *and* who live within 30 miles of a nuclear facility (11). While subsequent studies, such as Mangano in 2008, determined that African American infants in particular saw an increase in mortality after the Mississippi nuclear reactor, Grand Gulf, began operating, the Nuclear Regulatory Commission (NRC) has yet to alter Reference Man to reduce the levels of radiation emitted from the facilities (2).

Questions as to the relationship between nuclear facility emissions, low level doses of radiation, and health outcomes such as cancer are still contested as people residing near nuclear power facilities are more likely to be exposed to multiple environmental stressors, such as industrial/urban pollution, agricultural pesticides, herbicides, and fertilizer, and smoking. Currently, the National Academy of Sciences's Nuclear and Radiation Studies Board at the request of the NRC, is conducting an assessment of cancer risks near United States nuclear power facilities (12).

Regardless of the severity of the cancer risk, Executive Order 12898 may be being neglected. Further, the BEIR VII indicated that no level of radiation is safe for any child. To uphold the Order, we assessed if racial and socioeconomic disparities in children and families are associated with living in close proximity to an operating, licensed nuclear power plant. If the results are found to be positive, negative health outcomes are possible for the populations and we recommend to the NRC that Reference Man be reworked to protect the most vulnerable population: children.

In this study, we seek to assess if race and minority population-level characteristics for children and families are positively associated with living in close proximity to a nuclear power plant. This assessment will be conducted to determine if the definition for radiation protection standards, Reference Man, needs to be changed based on the population most likely to be exposed to radiation emitted from nuclear power plants. Previous domestic studies on nuclear power plants and environmental injustices have focused on the East Coast of the United States. Alldred and Shrader-Frechette examined the siting of nuclear facilities based on zip code-level data (6). Cousins et al. used mixed-methods to evaluate risks with a buffer calculated through an equation using seismic risk, spent fuel risk, and number of reactors as variables (4). Our study examines the impact region based on the recommendations provided by the National Cancer Institute as to the areas (Census block groups) with the greatest risk of developing cancer. To explicate the likelihood of minority and impoverished communities being exposed to low levels of ionizing radiation emitted from operating nuclear power plants, we compared the probability of living in close proximity to a nuclear power plant for those in the top tertile of minority and SES to the bottom tertile. Further, we explored if the likelihood of exposure for certain races was moderated by other race and SES characteristics. We used a multilevel logistic regression approach. The results of this study are relevant to the policy debate around reworking Reference Man.

OUR STUDY

The study area comprised 2010 US Census block groups in the following states: Alabama, Arkansas, Connecticut, Delaware, Florida, Georgia, Louisiana, Massachusetts, Maryland, Maine, North Carolina, New Hampshire, New Jersey, New York, Ohio, Pennsylvania, Rhode Island, South Carolina, Tennessee, Virginia, and West Virginia. The defined study area contained 104,635 block groups.

Nuclear power plant data

Locations of operating nuclear power plants were obtained from the Nuclear Regulatory Commission and Nuclear Tourist websites for 2010 (N = 36) (13, 14). We used ArcGIS 10.2 software to geocode the locations of all of these nuclear power plants against a 2010 Census block group map of the United States. We used a geographic information system (GIS) to create 30-mile buffers around each nuclear power plant to represent the area in which radiation levels could affect a person's health. Using the select by location query in ArcGIS, we identified block groups with their population centroid within 30-miles of a nuclear power plant. We defined proximity to a nuclear power plant in terms of a binary variable that equaled 1 if a given block group's centroid was within 30-miles of a nuclear power plant and 0 otherwise.

Demographic data

Using US Census data, we calculated at the census block group level the proportion of the population under 18 who were non-Hispanic black (proportion NHB) and the proportion of the population under 18 who were Hispanic (proportion Hispanic) (US Census Bureau, 2010), along with the proportion of families whose income in the past 12 months was below the poverty level (proportion in poverty) (15, 16). To allow for a nonlinear relationship between proximity to a nuclear power plant and each variable, we constructed tertiles of proportion NHB, proportion Hispanic, and proportion in poverty, corresponding to low (tertile 1), medium (tertile 2), and high (tertile 3) levels of each variable.

The analysis dataset was restricted to include only block groups with available data for race and SES across years (N = 103,517). We conducted multilevel logistic regression to model the association of proximity to a nuclear power plant with racial composition and poverty.

A state-level random intercept was included in all models to adjust standard errors for correlation among block groups within a given state. In the first three models, we estimated the unadjusted odds of proximity to a nuclear power plant associated with being in a higher tertile versus the first tertile for each race and poverty variable. The fourth model extended models 1-3 by including all race and poverty variables, thus estimating adjusted associations between race, poverty, and proximity to a nuclear power plant. The fifth model added all two-way interactions, and model 6 extended model 5 to include the three-way interaction among the racial composition variables and poverty.

Statistical significance of interactions terms was evaluated using nested likelihood ratio tests. Stratum-specific odds ratios (ORs) and associated 95% confidence intervals were estimated. All analyses were conducted in SAS 9.4 (SAS Institute, Cary NC) and R 3.1.1 (R Foundation for Statistical Computing, Vienna, Austria). Statistical significance was set at $\alpha = 0.05$.

FINDINGS

Race and poverty information were available for 103,517 block groups in the study area, including 22,868 block groups that were proximate to a nuclear power plant according to the 30-mile buffer definition.

In Table 1, block groups near to a nuclear power plant contained a higher average proportion Hispanic than those beyond the 30-mile buffer (16.49% versus 12.15%, respectively).

Table 1. Number of block groups with their population centroid within 30 miles and greater than 30 miles of nuclear power plant, and the corresponding average proportion NHB, Hispanic, and in poverty, Eastern United States (N = 103,517)

	All	Nuclear power plant within 30 miles	Nuclear power plant greater than 30 miles
N	103,517	22,868	80,649
%	100.00%	22.09%	77.91%
% NHB	20.77%	20.41%	20.87%
% Hispanic	13.11%	16.49%	12.15%
% in poverty	12.76%	12.05%	12.96%

Table 2. Proportion of block groups within 30 miles of a nuclear power plant by tertiles of proportion NHB, Hispanic, and in poverty (N = 103,517)

	% NHB			% Hispanic			% in poverty		
	Low % (n)	Medium % (n)	High % (n)	Low % (n)	Medium % (n)	High % (n)	Low % (n)	Medium % (n)	High % (n)
NPP within 30 miles	21.40% (7,385)	23.11% (7,974)	21.76% (7,509)	18.72% (6,461)	23.06% (7,961)	24.49% (8,446)	25.42% (8,775)	20.68% (7,135)	20.17% (6,958)
NPP greater than 30 miles	78.60% (27,123)	76.89% (26,259)	78.24% (26,997)	81.28% (28,046)	76.94% (26,556)	75.51% (26,047)	74.58 % (25,742)	79.32% (27,361)	79.83% (27,546)
Total	34,508	34,503	34,506	34,507	34,517	34,493	34,517	34,496	34,504

Low, medium, and high represent the following tertile categories: proportion NHB - < 2.68%, 2.68% - 18.43% and > 18.43%, proportion Hispanic - < 3.55%, 3.55% - 10.87%, and >10.87%, and proportion in poverty - < 3.66%, 3.66% - 14.15%, and >14.16%.

Table 3. Log odds coefficient estimates (betas) and 95% confidence intervals (CIs) in models of proximity to a nuclear power plant (N = 103,517)

	Tertile	Model 1 Beta (95% CI)	Model 2 Beta (95% CI)	Model 3 Beta (95% CI)	Model 4 Beta (95% CI)
% NHB	Low	0 [Reference]			0 [Reference]
	Medium	0.15*** (0.11, 0.19)			0.04* (-0.004, 0.08)
	High	0.15*** (0.10, 0.19)			0.08*** (0.03, 0.13)
% Hispanic	Low		0 [Reference]		0 [Reference]
	Medium		0.29*** (0.25, 0.33)		0.27*** (0.23, 0.32)
	High		0.44*** (0.40, 0.49)		0.46*** (0.41, 0.51)
% in poverty	Low			0 [Reference]	0 [Reference]
	Medium			-0.25*** (-0.30, -0.21)	-0.28*** (-0.33, -0.24)
	High			-0.16*** (-0.20, -0.12)	-0.25*** (-0.29, -0.20)
Intercept		-1.80 (-2.38, -1.23)	-1.93 (-2.49, -1.36)	-1.57 (-2.15, -1.00)	-1.79 (-2.35, -1.23)
Between state variation		1.75	1.69	1.76	1.65
LogLikelihood		-46579.2	-46418.3	-46528.7	-46306.1
Degrees of freedom (df)		4	4	4	8

Abbreviations: CI, confidence interval. * P < 0.1, ** P < 0.05, *** P < 0.01. Likelihood ratio tests comparing models 1, 2, 3, and 5 to model 4, respectively [$\chi^2, p-value$]: 546.23 (p < 0.001), 224.55 (p < 0.001), 445.2 (p < 0.001), 352.52 (p < 0.001). Likelihood ratio test comparing model 6 to model 5 [$\chi^2, p-value$]: 47.20 (p<0.001). Low, medium, and high represent the following tertile categories: proportion NHB - <2.68%, 2.68% - 18.43% and >18.43%, proportion Hispanic - <3.55%, 3.55% - 10.87%, and >10.87%, and proportion in poverty - <3.66%, 3.66% - 14.15%, and >14.16%.

Table 4. Stratum-specific odds ratios (ORs) and 95% confidence intervals (CIs) for close proximity to a nuclear power plant

	OR (95% CI) by tertiles of % Hispanic and % in poverty								
	% Hispanic low			% Hispanic medium			% Hispanic high		
% NHB	% in poverty low	% in poverty medium	% in poverty high	% in poverty low	% in poverty medium	% in poverty high	% in poverty low	% in poverty medium	% in poverty high
Low	1 [Reference]	1 [Reference]	1 [Reference]	1 [Reference]	1 [Reference]	1 [Reference]	1 [Reference]	1 [Reference]	1 [Reference]
Medium	1.10 (0.98, 1.26)	1.58*** (1.39, 1.81)	1.30** (1.04, 1.61)	1.02 (0.93, 1.11)	1.01 (0.91, 1.13)	1.28** (1.06, 1.55)	0.84*** (0.74, 0.95)	0.78*** (0.69, 0.89)	0.82** (0.70, 0.96)
High	0.81** (0.68, 0.97)	1.72*** (1.49, 1.98)	1.92*** (1.65, 2.25)	1.10 (0.97, 1.25)	1.14** (1.00, 1.29)	1.37*** (1.16, 1.62)	0.68*** (0.58, 0.78)	0.74*** (0.65, 0.85)	0.87* (0.75, 1.01)

	OR (95% CI) by tertiles of % NHB and % in poverty								
	% NHB low			% NHB medium			% NHB high		
% Hispanic	% in poverty low	% in poverty medium	% in poverty high	% in poverty low	% in poverty medium	% in poverty high	% in poverty low	% in poverty medium	% in poverty high
Low	1 [Reference]	1 [Reference]	1 [Reference]	1 [Reference]	1 [Reference]	1 [Reference]	1 [Reference]	1 [Reference]	1 [Reference]
Medium	1.09* (1.00, 1.19)	1.97*** (1.77, 2.20)	1.64*** (1.34, 2.00)	1.00 (0.89, 1.13)	1.26*** (1.10, 1.44)	1.62*** (1.32, 2.00)	1.48*** (1.22, 1.81)	1.30*** (1.12, 1.51)	1.17*** (1.05, 1.30)
High	1.41*** (1.25, 1.59)	2.96*** (2.58, 3.40)	3.53*** (2.91, 4.28)	1.07 (0.95, 1.21)	1.46*** (1.28, 1.67)	2.24*** (1.86, 2.69)	1.18* (0.97, 1.44)	1.28*** (1.10, 1.48)	1.60*** (1.46, 1.76)

	OR (95% CI) by tertiles of % NHB and % Hispanic								
	% NHB low			% NHB medium			% NHB high		
% in poverty	% Hispanic low	% Hispanic medium	% Hispanic high	% Hispanic low	% Hispanic medium	% Hispanic high	% Hispanic low	% Hispanic medium	% Hispanic high
Low	1 [Reference]	1 [Reference]	1 [Reference]	1 [Reference]	1 [Reference]	1 [Reference]	1 [Reference]	1 [Reference]	1 [Reference]
Medium	0.45*** (0.41, 0.50)	0.82*** (0.74, 0.91)	0.95 (0.31, 1.10)	0.65*** (0.56, 0.75)	0.82*** (0.74, 0.90)	0.88** (0.80, 0.98)	0.96 (0.78, 1.18)	0.84** (0.73, 0.97)	1.04 (0.91, 1.18)
High	0.39*** (0.34, 0.46)	0.59*** (0.51, 0.70)	0.98 (0.33, 1.17)	0.46*** (0.38, 0.56)	0.75*** (0.65, 0.85)	0.96 (0.87, 1.06)	0.93 (0.78, 1.12)	0.74*** (0.64, 0.84)	1.27*** (1.13, 1.42)

Abbreviations: OR, odds ratio; CI, confidence interval. * P < 0.1, ** P < 0.05, *** P < 0.01; Low, medium, and high represent the following tertile categories: proportion NHB - <2.68%, 2.68% - 18.43% and >18.43%, proportion Hispanic - <3.55%, 3.55% - 10.87%, and >10.87%, and proportion in poverty - <3.66%, 3.66% - 14.15%, and >14.16%.

The average proportion NHB and proportion in poverty did not appear to depend on proximity to a nuclear power plant. Almost a quarter of block groups characterized by high proportion Hispanic had a nuclear power plant nearby, an almost 6% increase compared to those characterized by low proportion Hispanic (see Table 2). About a quarter of block groups characterized by a low proportion in poverty were near a nuclear power plant, compared to 20.17% of those characterized by a high proportion in poverty.

Multilevel logistic regression analysis

Table 3 shows the estimated log-odds coefficients from the unadjusted and adjusted multilevel logistic regression models with no interactions. Across all models, tertiles of proportion NHB, proportion Hispanic, and proportion in poverty were significantly associated with close proximity to a nuclear power plant. Unadjusted models (models 1 through 3) indicated that block groups characterized by a medium or high proportion NHB or Hispanic were more likely to be in close proximity to a nuclear power plant compared to those characterized by a low proportion. In contrast, compared to block groups characterized by a low proportion in poverty, those characterized by a medium or high proportion in poverty were less likely to be in close proximity to a nuclear power plant. In the adjusted model with no interactions (model 4), the estimated log-odds coefficients did not substantively change, except for proportion NHB, which decreased in magnitude. Based on nested likelihood ratio tests, we found evidence of all two-way and three-way interactions (likelihood ratio test comparing model 6 to model 5: $\chi^2 = 47.20, p < 0.001$). As including the three-way interaction (model 6) resulted in an improved model fit, subsequent interpretation of stratum-specific associations will focus on model 6.

Non-Hispanic black and proximity to a nuclear power plant

Table 4 presents the stratum-specific odds ratios. Within the low Hispanic stratum, the odds of proximity to a nuclear power plant among block groups with a high versus low proportion NHB appeared to increase with increasing poverty. In fact, in the low Hispanic and low poverty stratum, high proportion NHB appeared protective (OR, 0.81; 95% CI, 0.68-0.97). In contrast, among block groups within the high Hispanic stratum, estimated ratios for high versus low proportion NHB appeared protective independent of poverty. Further, the estimated ratios for high and medium proportion NHB (compared to low proportion) were similar. In the medium Hispanic stratum, patterns in associations were less clear.

Hispanic and proximity to a nuclear power plant

Across NHB stratum, the odds of proximity to a nuclear power plant among block groups characterized by high versus low proportion Hispanic appeared to increase with increasing poverty. Interestingly, within the high NHB and low poverty stratum, the estimated odds of being proximate to a nuclear power plant among block groups characterized by a medium versus low proportion Hispanic (OR, 1.48; 95% CI, 1.22-1.81) were larger than the odds associated with a high versus low proportion Hispanic (OR, 1.18; 95% CI, 0.97-1.44).

SES and proximity to a nuclear power plant

Within the low NHB stratum, medium or high proportion in poverty appeared protective, except when proportion Hispanic was high. In fact, in the low NHB and low Hispanic stratum, a high proportion in poverty appeared very protective (OR, 0.39; 95% CI, 0.34-0.46), while in the low NHB and high Hispanic stratum, this protection waivered (OR, 0.98; 95% CI, 0.83-1.17).

Associations within the medium NHB stratum were similar, except when proportion Hispanic was high. When proportion Hispanic was high, a medium proportion in poverty appeared protective (OR, 0.88; 95% CI, 0.80-0.98). Within the high NHB stratum, estimated ratios for high versus low proportion in poverty appeared protective only when proportion Hispanic was medium. Further, within the high NHB and high Hispanic stratum, the estimated odds of being proximate to a nuclear power plant among block groups characterized by a high versus low proportion in poverty were 1.27 (95% CI, 1.13-1.42).

DISCUSSION

In the Eastern United States, certain impoverished and minority communities are at an increased risk of living in close proximity to a nuclear power plant. Communities with characteristics outside of those defined by Reference Man (white, male and young adult) are more likely to reside in close proximity to a nuclear power plant. Since all radiation emission standards are based upon Reference Man, the majority of the populations around nuclear power plants are not being protected. Thus, in order to protect those who are (a) most vulnerable to the effects of ionizing radiation and (b) most likely to reside in close proximity to a nuclear power plant, we recommend that Reference Man be redefined as Reference Most Vulnerable. Reference Most Vulnerable will ensure that the standard upon which radiation emissions levels are calculated will protect the health of all individuals regardless of their racial or socioeconomic background throughout the United States.

Our study was not without limitations. First, we used 2013 poverty data with 2010 racial composition data, as the American Community Survey replaced the census long form and the census no longer collects poverty or income information. Second, we looked at racial and SES disparities in the population surrounding operating nuclear power plants. As nuclear power plants that have been closed or decommissioned also emit low levels of ionizing radiation, it may be of interest in the future to include closed and decommissioned nuclear power plants in the study. Additionally, we did not take into account natural and built environmental effects or population count. Although we found block groups characterized by a high proportion NHB to be protective when proportion Hispanic and proportion in poverty were concentrated, this may speak to confounding caused by urban/rural status, as large cities not in close proximity to a nuclear power plant contain areas of concentrated poverty and minority status.

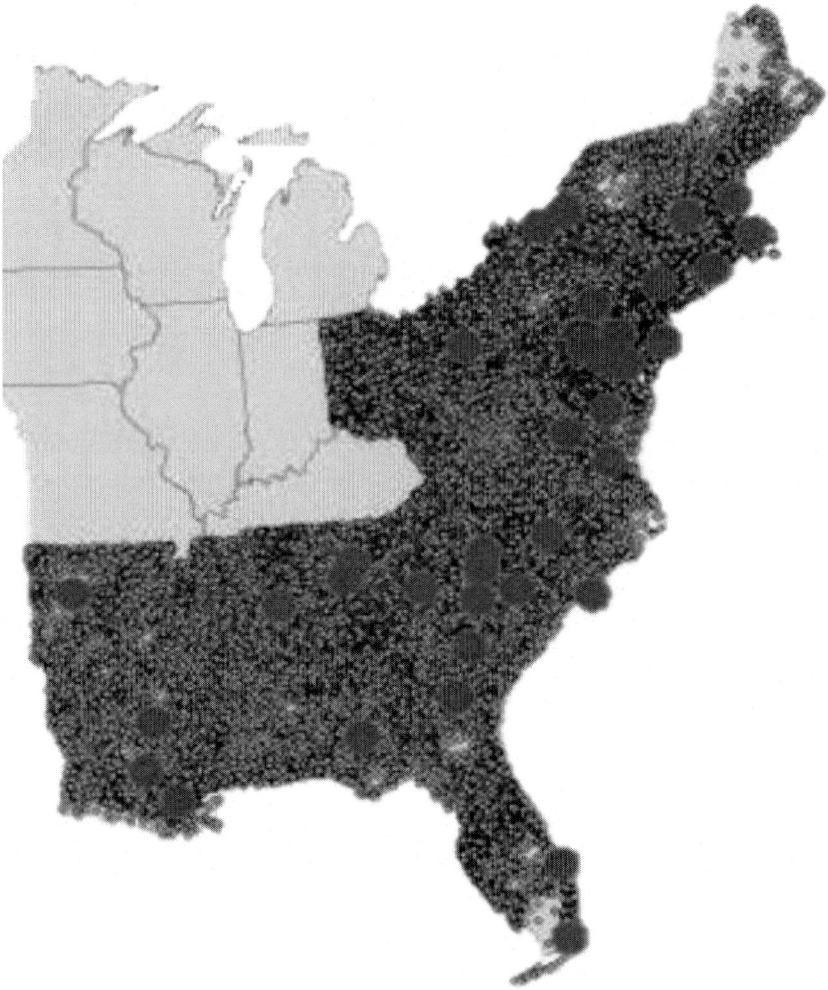

Figure 1. Eastern United States block groups located within a 30-mile buffer of a nuclear power plant. Generated using ArcMap 10.1.1.

Further studies should examine this relationship by urban rural status. Due to certain block groups being located in large cities that contain concentrated areas of high disadvantage and high proportion minority, our next step is to perform an analysis stratified by rural and urban areas. Finally, future studies should consider whether the 30-mile buffer zone encompasses all individuals exposed to low levels of ionizing radiation and if the individual level would be more precise.

In conclusion, although our study was limited, it does elucidate a flaw in the current radiation protection standards. Our results suggest that certain disadvantaged and minority communities in the Eastern United States are at an increased risk of being located near a nuclear power plant, indicating that these communities are also at an increased risk of being exposed to low levels of radiation emitted from a nuclear power plant. As the current radiation protection standard is based on a white, adult male, Reference Man should be expanded to consider characteristics of the most vulnerable in these impoverished and minority communities.

ACKNOWLEDGMENTS

The preparation for this paper and project were supported Rebecca Anthopolos and Nicki Sandberg of the Children's Environmental Health Initiative at the University of Michigan's School of Natural Resources and Environment.

REFERENCES

[1] Bullard R. Unequal protection: Environmental justice and communities of color. San Francisco, CA: Sierra Club Books, 1997.

[2] Mangano J. Excess infant mortality after nuclear plant startup in rural Mississippi. Int J Hlth Serv 2008;38(2).

[3] Gray S, Edwards S. Miranda M. Race, socioeconomic status, and air pollution exposure in North Carolina. Environ Res 2013;126:152-8.

[4] Cousins E, Karban C, Li F, Zapanta M. Nuclear power and environmental justice: A mixed-methods study of risk, vulnerability, and the victim experience. Comprehensive exercise. Carelton, MN: Carleton College, 2013.

[5] Sherman D. Critical mechanisms for critical masses: Exploring variation in opposition to low-Level radioactive waste site proposals. Mobilization 2011;16(1):81-100.

[6] Alldred M, Shrader-Frechette K. Environmental injustice in siting nuclear plants. Environ Just 2009;2:1-11.

[7] Sermage-Faure C, Lauroier D, Goujon-Bellec S, Chartier M, Guyot-Goubin A, Rudant J, et al. Childhood leukemia around French nuclear power plants: The Geocap study, 2002-2007". Int J Cancer 2012;131(5):E769-80.

[8] Kaatsch P, Spix C, Jung I, Blettner M. Childhood leukemia in the vicinity of nuclear power plants in Germany. Deutsches Arzteblatt Int 2008;105(42):725-32.

[9] Jablon S. Cancer in populations living near nuclear facilities. JAMA 1990;265:1403.

[10] National Academy of Sciences. Health risks from exposure to low levels of ionizing radiation: BEIR VII Phase 2. Washington, DC: National Academies Press, 2006.

[11] Makhijani A, Smith B. Thorne M. Science for the vulnerable setting radiation and multiple exposure environmental health standards to protect those most at risk. Takoma Park, MD: Institute Energy Environmental Research, 2006:1-107.

[12] National Academy of Sciences. Analysis of cancer risks in populations near nuclear facilities. URL: http://nas sites.org/cancerriskstudy/

[13] Nuclear Regulatory Commission. Operating nuclear power reactors by location or name, Updated 2015. URL: http://www.nrc.gov/info-finder/reactor/.

[14] Gonyeau J. The virtual nuclear tourist, 2011. URL: http://www.nucleartourist.com.

[15] United States Census Bureau. 2010 Census, 2011. URL: http://www.census.gov/2010census.

[16] United States Census Bureau. 2013 population estimates, 2013. URL: http://www.census.gov/.

In: Environmental Health Disparities
Editors: I Leslie Rubin and Joav Merrick

ISBN: 978-1-63484-211-2

Chapter 5

ASTHMA AND AFRICAN-AMERICAN CHILDREN IN LOW-INCOME COMMUNITIES

Jasmine Williams and Saul Mofya**, DVM, MSc
Department of Veterinary Science and Public Health,
Fort Valley State University, Fort Valley, Georgia, US

The prevalence of asthma in the United States is steadily increasing, affecting African-Americans and Latino groups more significantly. In this chapter we conducted a literature review to established health disparities and factors that trigger asthma in African-American children in low-income communities in Fort Valley, GA. Review of the literature shows that triggering factors contributing to the high prevalence, severity and poorer health outcomes of childhood asthma in African-American communities include a variety of socioeconomic factors, such as poverty, low literacy, health behaviors, lack of access to health care and access to health insurance, housing structures, and environmental exposures. We propose that, in order to break the cycle of health disparities and factors that trigger asthma, a partnership involving community leaders, medical, environmental, and public health professionals creates a forum to promote asthma awareness in order to empower members of the community to address the factors adversely impacting their health. Mobilizing a diverse group of stakeholders and focusing on health and education policy and system which addresses disparities in both health and education should be a top priority in low-income communities. The recruiting of culturally diverse and culturally competent health professionals and practice leadership should be a common goal. Strategies within the control of the community can be taught to improve safety and promote better health practices. Additional activities towards improving education and reducing health disparities could include raising funds and support to renovate housing units which are in a dilapidated state, and to provide more community based health literacy training.

* Correspondence: Assistant Professor Saul Mofya, DVM, MSc, Department of Veterinary Science and Public Health, Fort Valley State University, Fort Valley, Georgia, United States. E-mail: mofyas@fvsu.edu.

INTRODUCTION

Asthma is the most common chronic disease among United States children and the leading cause of childhood morbidity. The disease disproportionately burdens many socioeconomically disadvantaged communities, especially in urban cities (1). The Centers of Disease Control and Prevention (CDC) estimates that there are over 25.5 million people with asthma in the United States and approximately one third of these are children (1). Despite effective therapies, asthma prevalence, morbidity, and mortality among children is increasing in the United States, largely affecting minority and low-income groups. African- American and Latino children who live in low-socioeconomic-status within urban environments have been shown in some studies to be the most affected (2, 3).

Several studies have concluded that, as with many chronic conditions, disparities in asthma outcomes may be due to factors such as race, socioeconomic status(SES), housing, environmental exposure, low parental literacy, health insurance, quality of health care, and/or differing self-management strategies (2, 3). According to a study by researchers at John Hopkins University, African-Americans had more severe symptoms than any other racial or ethnic group yet lacked the necessary information about avoiding asthma triggers (1). This study indicated that African-Americans were three to four times more likely than Caucasians to be hospitalized for asthma, and were four to six times more likely to die from this disease. They were also less likely to receive treatment, which contributes to the problem (1).

The purpose of this study was to assess health disparities and factors that trigger asthma in African-American children in low-income communities in Fort Valley, Georgia and to provide recommendations that may assist medical and public health professionals and other stakeholders to educate these communities.

LITERATURE REVIEW

To assess health disparities and factors that trigger asthma in African-American children in low-income communities in Fort Valley, we conducted literature reviews which included the North Central Health District Peach County 2013 Health Status Report, Community Health Needs Assessment Peach Country 2015, the city-data of Fort Valley, GA, and several peer reviewed articles relating to our search.

FINDINGS

Fort Valley is a city in Peach County, Georgia. The current total population for Peach County is 27,481, composed of predominantly Caucasians (47.26%) and African-Americans (46.5%) (4). However, the current population in the city of Fort Valley is estimated to be 10,000 people, 81% being African-Americans (5).

Asthma prevalence

According to the North Central Health District Peach County 2013 Health Status Report, from 2006-2010 in Peach County asthma accounted for 789 (1.3%) emergency department visits and had a hospital discharge rate of 154.9 per 100,000.

Children ages 1-12 were most affected by asthma symptoms that led to an emergency department visit. The emergency department visit rates in Peach County due to asthma were much higher for African-Americans (974.9 per 100,000 people) and other races (489 per 100,000 people) compared to Caucasians (253.9 per 100,000 people) (6).

Socioeconomic status (SES)

The median household income in Fort Valley per year is $ 24,661; for the State of Georgia it is $ 49,604, while the national average is $53,046. Fort Valley has an unemployment rate (11.8%) which is above state 6.8% and the national average of 6.0%. It is estimated that 36% of the children live in poverty, more than 70% of the students are on free or reduced lunch, and 19% of the households are on food stamp/SNAP benefits (6).

Education status

Only 21.3% of our target population are functionally illiterate, with an average high school graduation rate of less than 60% (6).

Housing

The majority of the housing units in the area were built in the 1960s and are in deplorable condition. Over 34% of housing units are classified as substandard because they have at least one of the following conditions: 1) lacking complete plumbing facilities, 2) lacking complete kitchen facilities, 3) having more than 1 occupant per room (4).

Health behaviors

Health behaviors such as poor diet, a lack of exercise, and tobacco smoking contribute to poor health status. 27.8% of the adults lack exercise, 34.6% are obese and 20.2 % are current tobacco users (6). Half of the restaurants in the area are fast food establishments. Because current behaviors are determinants of future health, these indicators may predispose to future significant health issues, such as poor cardiovascular health and other complications of obesity such as diabetes (4,6).

Health insurance

22.4% of the adults and 8.2% of children do not have health insurance (6).

Environmental exposure

Fort Valley tends to experience high temperatures and humidity, which are above the national average (5). These environmental factors are favorable for mold growth, which is one of the known triggering factors for asthma attacks. The area is ranked 14th in the nation as a city where people are at risk of year-round air particle pollution (5).

Discussion

This study sought to determine health disparities and factors that trigger asthma in African-American children in low-income communities in Fort Valley, Georgia.

Socioeconomic status

Poverty has been directly and indirectly associated with health disparities and severity of illnesses. African-American populations with low SES, whether measured based on income or occupation have higher levels of illness than populations with higher income (2). Numerous studies have shown that mortality rates in almost every illness, including asthma, are higher in African-American populations with low SES than those seen in Caucasians or other groups with higher SES (2,3). From our literature review, the majority of African-American families in Fort Valley live in neighborhoods where 44% of families' income is below the Federal poverty level. This percentage is more than three times the national level (4).

Families and individuals with low SES are more likely to engage in high-risk behaviors associated with asthma exacerbations, such as smoking tobacco and illicit substances, eating fast foods more frequently or not exercising (6). In the United States, tobacco smoking and environmental tobacco smoking (Second hand tobacco exposure) vary widely by socioeconomic status and ethnicity (7). Current tobacco smoking in adults in Fort Valley is 20.2%, while the national rate is 18.1% (4, 6). Exposure of children or pregnant women to environmental tobacco smoke predisposes toward both earlier onset and increased severity of asthma. Maternal smoking in pregnancy may influence the development of the fetal respiratory system as well as lung function impairment in newborns (8). Several studies have concluded that maternal smoking in pregnancy increases the risk of asthma during the early part of the child's life. Smoking also contributes to low birth weight and preterm delivery, which are independent determinants of asthma (8). As for our study area, environmental tobacco smoking is a major concern as children are exposed both in homes and neighborhood communities. The need to start promoting and sensitizing the communities about the detrimental effect of tobacco smoking on the general health of the community should be a priority.

The prevalence of obesity and asthma in United States has increased drastically over the past 20 years (9). Epidemiologic studies have shown that obesity serves as a modifier for asthma risk (10). From our literature review, 27.8% of the adults lack exercise and 34.6% are obese (4, 6); this finding also may apply to the children in these communities. Lack of exercise and obesity can be attributed to health behaviors which are associated with low SES and poor diet. Notably, 50% of restaurant establishments in Fort Valley are fast foods. Eating excessive fast foods combined with a sedentary lifestyle predispose to obesity. Obese children are at an increased risk of experiencing severe asthma symptoms (11). There is a strong relationship between obesity and asthma, both of which show increasing prevalence.

According to asthma surveillance data from the Centers for Disease Control and Prevention (CDC), as recently as 2013, the prevalence of asthma in children in the United States was 8.3% and data from National Health and Nutrition Examination Survey (NHANES), put the prevalence of obesity in youth nearly 17%. It has been noted that both obesity and asthma affect certain minority and inner-city groups more than other populations (10, 11). In addition, it appears that even a little excess weight can directly affect lung function, particularly in minority children (11).

Childhood obesity can have complications for child's physical, social, and emotional well-being. Obese children are exposed to weight stigma and are vulnerable to psychological effects, such as depression, and social effects, such as isolation. Consequences of bias, such as isolation or social withdrawal, could contribute to the exacerbation of obesity through psychological vulnerabilities that increase the likelihood of over-eating and sedentary activity (3, 11).

Access to health care

Many African-American populations tend to access health care in fewer numbers compared to Caucasians. The reason varies from lack of health insurance to established beliefs and biases about interactions between African-Americans and their health care providers (12, 13). The predominant barriers include inability to pay for services, lack of health insurance, lack of transportation and child care, decreased understanding of treatment plans and inability to incorporate prescribed health plans into daily living patterns (2, 14). Furthermore, some African- American populations' cultural beliefs and health practices have a significant impact upon their well-being regardless of their income and educational levels (13).

Various health beliefs and practices can be observed among African-American groups, in part determined by their ages, socioeconomic levels and geographic locales. However, common cultural threads can be identified among many African-Americans. These commonalities include religious orientation, social support networks, and informal health care system (13). Religion is a central force within the lives of many African-Americans. Religious beliefs influence all aspects of many African-American families and communities' lives, including work, education, recreation and health. Health is not viewed as made up of physiological and psychological components as defined within the traditional science oriented framework of health; rather, the beliefs of many African-American characterizes health as a continuum evolving around mind, body, and spirit 13. Many African-Americans are more likely to use prayer as a means of coping with worries than Caucasians peers (13) rather than seeking professional help, which is sorely limited anyway.

Support systems which are often utilized by African-Americans have a significant role in the lives of individuals. These support system include significant others who may or may not be related by blood or marriage. In times of crisis and stress, African-Americans are more likely to rely on the family network, both nuclear and extended than on outside traditional health and human service community agencies (13).

Informal health- care systems within the African-American community are often consulted. In the event of illness African-Americans are more likely to consult family members and friends than the professional health-care system (13).

Cultural values often influence the degree of adherence to health care treatment regimes. A number of studies have also shown that, in the African-American populations studied, at least a third of the patients would not take prescribed medicines due to cultural and health beliefs (13). In addition, lack of communication and understanding between patients and providers has also been a major contributing factor to asthma health disparities (14). Low literacy levels have been found within Fort Valley communities. In communities similar to Fort Valley, low literacy can contribute to misunderstanding information and directions provided by the physician. One study found that physicians seeing African-American patients would more likely control the conversation and talk to them less about their conditions compared to physicians seeing Caucasian patients (14). Health professionals need a particular skill set in order to provide culturally competent health care to minority patients, families and communities. Health professionals bemoan the lack of time, resources, and/or information to do so, yet they fail to recognize that these are the same reasons offered by patients who have difficulties managing a recommended therapeutic regimen.

Health insurance

We found that more than 8.2% of children and 22.4% of adults lack health insurance coverage (6). The percentage of children and adult lacking health insurance at national level is 7.5% and 15% respectively (4). More than 90% of children who have health insurance in Fort Valley have it with Medicaid or the State Children's Health Insurance Program. While Medicaid may improve access to care for low SES children who are otherwise uninsured, it does not ensure their access to the same locations and providers of care, nor the same continuity of care that children with private insurance receive (1). Choice among providers may be significantly limited in locations where the Medicaid provider payment rate is low compared to other insurers.

In Peach County, the emergency department visit rates due to asthma were much higher for African-American children, especially those between the ages of 1-12 years (6). Parents in these communities may only take their children to the emergency department when they show severe symptoms of an asthma exacerbation. These seek medical relief rather than treatment and control of the disease, perhaps due to the general complexities related to the health insurance enrollment process, lack of money to pay for medical services, and to some extent lack of transportation (14). Furthermore, complex enrollment rules and processes for initial enrollment and maintaining enrollment in Medicaid are commonly noted, compromising child participation in this program (2).

Housing structure

Housing- poor or substandard housing units are more likely to have above average exposure to indoor allergens, such as dust mites, rodent allergens, cockroach allergens, mold and mildew (8, 12). In the Fort Valley area, most of the houses were built in the 1960s and are now in dilapidated condition, which contribute to indoor allergens.

Several epidemiological studies have linked substandard housing with an increased risk of chronic illness. Damp, cold, and moldy housing is associated with asthma and other chronic respiratory symptoms, even after potentially confounding factors such as income, socioeconomic status; smoking, crowding, and unemployment are controlled (16, 17). Water intrusion is a major contributor to problems with dampness. The dilapidated condition of many homes in Fort Valley area makes it likely that they have both interior and exterior leaks. Overcrowding and inadequate ventilation also increase interior moisture. Damp houses provide a nurturing environment for mites, roaches, respiratory viruses, and molds, all of which play a role in respiratory disease pathogenesis (12). Cross-sectional epidemiological studies have also established associations between damp and moldy housing and recurrent headaches, fever, nausea and vomiting, and sore throats (8, 18, 19).

Old, dirty carpeting, often found in substandard housing, is a significant reservoir for dust, allergens, and toxic chemicals (12). Exposure to these agents can result in allergic, respiratory, neurological, and hematologic illnesses. Pest infestations, through their association with asthma, provide another linkage between substandard housing and chronic illness (17). Cockroaches can cause allergic sensitization and have emerged as an important asthma trigger in inner-city neighborhoods (8). Children with asthma who are sensitized and exposed to cockroaches are at elevated risk for hospitalization (8). Mouse allergen also acts as a clinically important cause of allergy and asthma morbidity (8). Structural defects in substandard housing permit entry of cockroaches and rodents; leaking pipes and other sources of water provide them with water to drink. Inadequate food storage and disposal facilities provide pests with opportunities for obtaining food. Dead spaces in walls harbor pests and permit circulation among apartments in multiunit dwellings (17).

Minority children are significantly more likely to be exposed to indoor allergens as well as second hand smoke, which is a known contributor to asthma prevalence and morbidity (1). Our literature review indicted that 20.2% of the adults are current tobacco smokers (6). Unfortunately, most of these smokers also smoke indoors, exacerbating indoor air quality.

Environmental factors

A significant factor that contributes to asthma is air pollution. Air pollutants are associated with a high incidence of asthma attacks, as well as morbidity of respiratory illness (20). Fort Valley is ranked 14th in the nation as a city where people are at risk of year-round air particle pollution.

In Peach county (where Fort Valley is located), the average daily ambient Particulate Matter (PM2.5) is 11.9$\mu g/m^3$ with 5 days exceeding emissions standards while the national average PM2.5 is 10.7$\mu g/m^3$ with four days exceeding emissions standards (4). While the PM2.5 for Fort Valley is within acceptable range, individuals that are particularly sensitive to fine particle exposure (such as those with heart or lung disease, older adults, and children) can experience severe symptoms (20). It is also important to understand that concentration of particulate matter in indoor air can differ substantially from outdoor concentrations. When substandard housing results in poor ventilation and low air exchange rates, contributions from indoor particulate sources such as cooking appliances and heaters can accumulate to dangerous levels (21).

Other factors that may contribute to air pollution in the area include diesel exhaust from large trucks, cargo trains, and a school bus assembly plant, as well as agricultural pesticides. Diesel exhaust emissions contribute to the development and exacerbation of asthma, because of both the numerous chemical irritants and the large volume of small particulate matter (21). Peach County is one of the largest producers of peaches in Georgia, facilitated by the common place use of agricultural pesticides by farmers. Most of the pesticides are aerosols and can trigger allergies, asthma and respiratory irritation, especially in children and elderly. These pollutants have been known to increase airway obstruction, resulting in a greater number of children being hospitalized in these polluted areas (21).

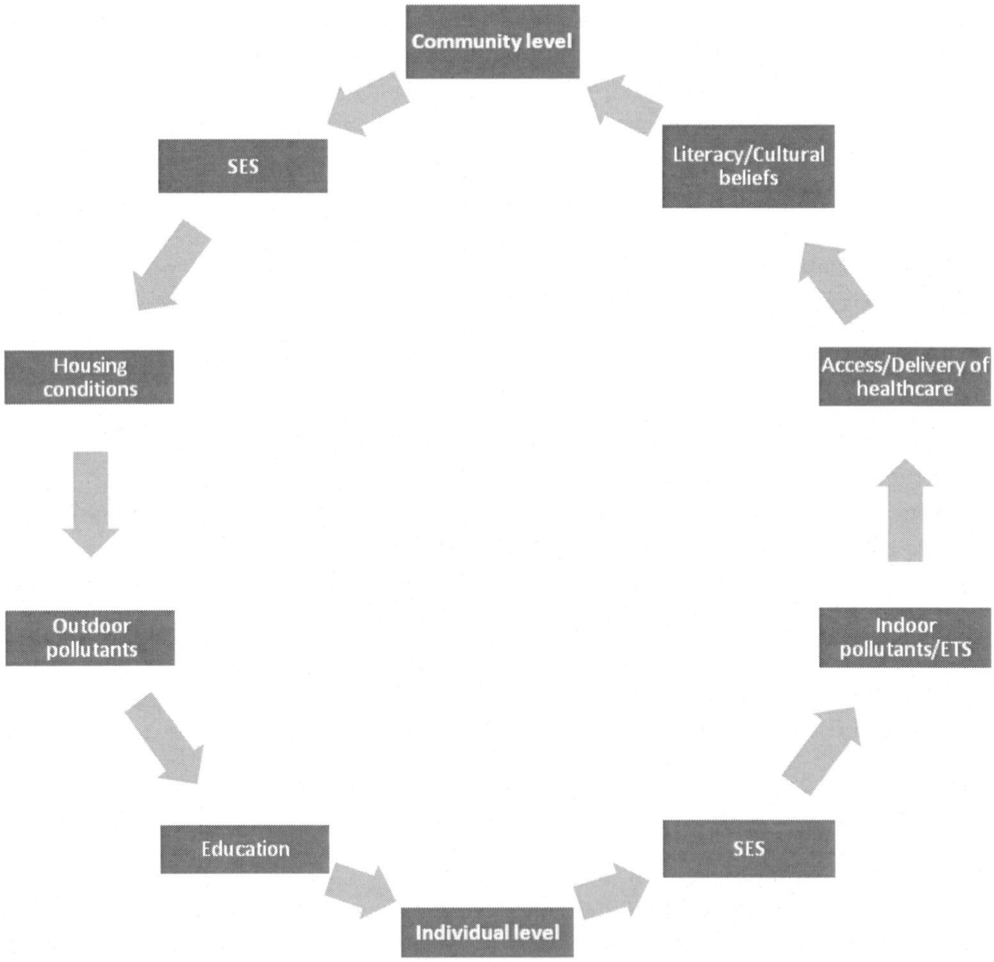

Figure 1. Known determinants of asthma disparities.

The weather in the area also plays a major role in contributing to asthma exacerbations in the children. Fort Valley tends to experience hot and humid conditions in the summer months, with temperatures and humidity above the national average levels (5). The temperature ranges from 45-95 degree Fahrenheit, with humidity of 50 to 90% throughout the year. The national temperature and humidity ranges from 30-90 degree Fahrenheit and 40-80% respectively (5). Such environmental conditions, coupled with substandard or dilapidated housing units, encourage the growth of mold and mildew which are well known factors that triggers asthma (17, 22). Figure 1 shows the cycle of environmental health disparities and known determinants of asthma in Fort Valley. In order to break the cycle, several measures need to be considered. We suggested some of the important ways to break the cycle in the conclusion section of this article.

Conclusion

Our survey of the literature recognized factors which contribute to health disparities and asthma triggers in African-American children in low-income communities in Fort Valley. These factors include SES, (low literacy, health behaviors, limited access to health care, and lack of health insurance), dilapidated housing structures, and environmental exposure. Issues with SES include poverty, tobacco smoking, obesity, and increased risk of low quality health care due to problems, which originate from established beliefs and issues of communication between patient and provider. Environmental factors include indoor allergens, the condition of housing, weather conditions, and air pollution. One potential strategy to address these complex and compounding health issues is to forge a collaborative partnership between community leaders, medical, environmental, and public health professionals to promote asthma awareness in communities and schools.

The most important step to address the asthma disparities in Fort Valley would be to implement and enforce policies that increase access to healthcare for children and adults with asthma, regardless of their ethnicity or SES. This can be achieved through affordable health insurance with an easy enrollment system. If the enrollment system cannot be simplified, community-based enrollment programs should be implemented to help people to navigate through the complex health insurance system.

Access to high quality health care is essential. High quality health care involves culturally competent care, and ensures that patients receive high-quality, effective care irrespective of cultural background, language proficiency, socio-economic status and other factors that may be formed by a patient's race or ethnicity. Lack of cultural awareness can undermine the physician-patient relationship. Providers should ensure that patients receive effective, understandable, respectful care compatible with cultural and linguistic preferences. The recruiting of culturally diverse and culturally competent staff and practice leadership should be a common goal. High quality care also involves delivering patient-centered care which emphasizes respect for the patient, clear communication, shared decision making, and building of the physician-patient relationship.

Health status is influenced not only by access to health care but also by socioeconomic determinants, such as income and availability of nutritious foods, environmental health of the community and access to early childhood education. Stakeholders and policymakers must also address these factors that play a part influencing the health of African-Americans and minority communities.

An individual's socioeconomic status, particularly income and education level, is among the many factors that significantly influence health. Lower-income individuals, regardless of race or ethnicity, are often in poorer health than those in higher income brackets. An individual's income may influence a number of other determinants of health status, such as one's access to educational opportunities, decent medical care, and affordable housing in a healthy community. A person's level of education also affects health status. Therefore, education is critical to increase the likelihood of employment and of better income that breaks the cycle.

Increased emphasis must be placed on reducing disparities in education if the health disparity gap is to be closed. Investments in early childhood education and after-school programs for underserved minorities should be made to ensure academic success later in life. Evidence shows that minority children who attended early childhood education program are less likely than those not to engage in high-risk activities, such as smoking and illicit drug use (23). In addition, children who regularly attended after-school programs have markedly increased academic performance compared with students who are unsupervised after school (23).

Physical fitness education is even more important, to combat the increasingly sedentary habits of young children. School and community based physical activities should be encouraged in these communities, such as swimming, marathon, cycling and several outdoor games.

A number of significant barriers impede the growth of African-Americans and other minority students in health professions. Among the greatest impediments faced by racial and ethnic minorities is unequal access to adequate educational opportunities and parental inability to access costly private-sector substitutes even if these are available. African-Americans and other minorities often are caught in the "Cycle of disadvantage and disability": often educated at schools with insufficient financial resources, less-qualified teaching staff, and fewer advanced courses, contributing to lower academic achievement. This lack of educational preparedness poses a challenge to students hoping to enter the medical professions. African- Americans and other minorities are disproportionately low-income and are often educated at schools with insufficient financial resources, less-qualified teaching staff, and fewer advanced courses. The need to improve educational opportunities for all children through local, state and federal funding should be a top priority if the health and education disparity gap is to be closed.

Public health education campaigns and programs targeting high- risk groups should be utilized to educate citizens about healthy living, the importance of prevention, and risk factors that contribute to preventable illness. These campaigns and programs should be community-driven to ensure that the materials and messages are tailored to the needs of the local population and reflect the culture of the community.

Efforts must be made to reduce the effect of environmental stressors that disproportionately threaten to harm the health and well-being of low-SES communities. An individual's environment can have a significant impact on his or her overall health status. Environmental dangers, such as poor air quality, mold growth or rampant lead contamination can harm the health of the community. Substandard housing is a likely contributor to the elevated rate of exposure to environmental stressors, as these homes are more likely to be located close to noxious land use such as industrial sites or hazardous dumping areas. Addressing health disparities that are the effect of environmental stressors is a complex and difficult task. However, more action needs to be taken to address, rectify and monitor the harmful effect of environmental stressors on minority communities.

In conclusion, methods that the families are capable of carrying out can also be taught to make communities health and safer. Activities such as fundraisers to raise money to renovate housing units which are dilapidated, community gardening and providing more family based program including nutrition and diet, exercise and smoking cessation are needed in order to lower asthma rates in low-income communities.

REFERENCES

[1] Akinbami LJ, Moorman JE, Bailey C, Zahran HS, King M, Johnson CA, et al. Treads in asthma prevalence, health care use and mortality in the united States,2001-2010. NCHS Data Brief 2012;94: 1-8.

[2] Neeta TN, Oh SS, Nguyen EA, Martin M, Roth LA, Galanter J, et al. Socioeconomic status and childhood asthma in urban minority youths. The GALA II and SAGE II studies. Am J Respir Crit Care Med 2013;188(10):1202-9.

[3] Carroll K. Socioeconomic status, race/ethnicity and asthma in youth. Am J Respir Crit Care Med 2013;188:1180-1.

[4] Georgia Department of Health. Georgia, Peach County. Full health indicators report. Community health needs assessment. North Central Health District. Fort Valley, GA: Peach County Health Department, 2015.

[5] Fort Valley, Georgia. City-Data.com. URL: www.city-data.com/city/Fort-Valley-Georgia.

[6] Georgia Department of Public Health. 2013 North Central Health District, Peach County: Health status report. Fort Valley, GA: Georgia Department Public Health, 2014.

[7] Kit BK, Simon AE, Brody DJ, Akinbami LJ. US prevalence and tread in tobacco smoke exposure among children and adolescents with asthma. Pediatrics 2013;131(3):407-14.

[8] Kanchongkittiphon W, Gaffin JM, Phipatanakul W The indoor environment and inner-city childhood asthma. Asian Pac J Immunol 2014; 32:103-10.

[9] Wang Y. Disparities in pediatric obesity in the United States. Am Soc Nutr Adv Nutr 2011;2:23-31.

[10] Dooyema CA, Belay B, Foltz JL, Williams N, Blanck HM. The childhood obesity research demonstration project: A comprehensive community approach to reduce childhood obesity. Childhood Obes 2013;9(5):454-9.

[11] Quinto KB, Zuraw BL, Poon KY, Chen W, Schatz M, Christiansen SC. The association of obesity and asthma severity and control in children. J Allergy Clin Immunol 2011;128(5):964-9.

[12] Holt EW, Theall KP, Rabito FA. Individual, housing and neighborhood correlates of asthma among young urban children. J Urban Hlth 2013;90: 116-29.

[13] George M. Health beliefs,treatment preferences and complementary and alternative medicine for asthma, smoking and lung cancer self-management in diverse black communities. Patient Educ Couns 2012;89(3):489-500.

[14] Perry TT, Rettiganti M, Brown RH, Nick TG, Jones SM. Uncontrolled asthma and factors related to morbidity in an impoverished, rural environment. Ann Allergy Asthma Immunol 2012;108(4):254-9.

[15] Cabana MD, Slish KK, Evans D, Mellins RB, Brown RW, Lin X, et al. Impact of physician asthma care education on patient outcomes. Pediatrics 2006;117(6):2149-57.

[16] Breysse J, Dixon S, Gregory J, Philby M, Jacobs DE, Krieger J. Effect of weatherization combined with community health worker in-home education on asthema control. Am J Publ Hlth 2014;104(1):57-64.

[17] Turyk M, Banda E, Chisum G, Weems D Jr, Liu Y, Damitz M, et al. A multifaceted community-based asthma intervention in Chicago:effects of trigger reduction and self-management education on asthma morbidity. J Asthma 2013;50(7):727-36.

[18] Strachan DP. Damp housing and childhood asthma: Validation of reporting of symptoms. BMJ 1988;297:1223-6.

[19] Institute of Medicine. Damp indoor spaces and health. Washington, DC: National Academies Press, 2004.

[20] Lewis TC, Robins TG, Mentz GB, Zhang X, Mukherjee B, Lin X, et al. Air pollution and respiratory symptoms among children with asthma:Vulnerability by corticosteroid use and residence area. Sci Total Environ 2013;448:48-55.

[21] Adamkiewicz G, Zota AR, Fabian MP, Chahine T, Julien R, Spengler JD, et al. Moving environmental justice indoors: Understanding structural influences on residential exposure patterns in low-income communities. Am J Publ Health 2011;101(Suppl 1):s238-45.

[22] Meng YY, Babey SH, Wolstein J. Asthma-related school absenteeism and school concentration of low-income students in California. Prev Chronic Dis 2012; 9:1103-12.

[23] American College of Physicians. Racial and ethnic disparities in health care. Philadelphia, PA: American College Physicians, 2010.

In: Environmental Health Disparities
Editors: I Leslie Rubin and Joav Merrick

ISBN: 978-1-63484-211-2

Chapter 6

IMPACT OF HOUSING ON PUBERTAL TIMING

Farah Dadabhoy[1,*], MSc, Maida Galvez[2], MD, Ashley Pajak[2], MSc, Susan Teitelbaum[2], PhD, and Mary Wolff[2], PhD

[1]University of Cincinnati College of Medicine,
Cincinnati, Ohio, US

[2]Department of Preventive Medicine and Pediatrics,
Icahn School of Medicine at Mount Sinai,
New York, US

This chapter explores the associations between housing quality and timing of puberty in urban Black and Hispanic girls. Methods: Black and Hispanic girls living in New York City, ages 6 to 8 years (n = 416), were enrolled in a longitudinal study, Growing Up Healthy. After 8 years, we had information on housing and puberty stages for 331 girls. Interviews administered to guardians gathered information on caregiver education and whether they lived in public or private housing. Stages of breast and pubic hair development and body mass index (BMI) were assessed annually by pediatric providers and trained field staff. Overall, BMI and pubertal stages (any breast development [stage B2+] vs none, and pubic hair, any vs none) were examined in relation to housing, race/ethnicity, and caregiver education. Results: Forty percent of the cohort was overweight irrespective of housing. The proportion of girls having earlier B2+ was similar among Black and Hispanic girls regardless of housing type. Pubic hair development occurred earlier in Hispanic girls living in public housing compared to those living in private housing ($p < 0.01$, adjusted for BMI and caregiver education). Among Hispanic girls, 48% of those living in private housing began pubic hair development before 10 years old whereas 79% of those living in public housing began pubic hair development before 10 years old. Conclusion: Preliminary unadjusted analyses suggest a potential role for housing type on development of puberty in girls. Housing quality may be associated with earlier age of pubic hair growth in Hispanic girls.

* Correspondence: Farah Dadabhoy, 231 MLK Dr. E, Apt 6, Cincinnati, Ohio 45219, United States. E-mail: fzdadabhoy@gmail.com.

INTRODUCTION

For the past several decades, the timing of puberty has been the subject of debate. Typically, puberty in girls is characterized by certain momentous transitions. It begins with breast development, followed by the appearance of pubic and axillary hair, a growth spurt, finally culminating in menstruation. As research continues to pursue this tumultuous process, there is mounting consensus that key pubertal milestones, specifically breast and pubic hair development, are presenting earlier in a girl's life (1-7). Recent epidemiological studies find that by age 8 years approximately 43% of Black girls, 31% of Hispanic girls and 18% of White girls have exhibit breast development (2). Consequently, an increasing number of families are forced to confront the social and physical challenges of puberty, before they may be prepared to do so.

While obesity is frequently implicated as the leading cause of early puberty, novel insights in the field emphasize that increases in body size and weight account for only part of the decline in pubertal age (8-12). Increasingly, environmental and lifestyle factors are now a focus of study. One study (13), which tracked over two thousand girls in Copenhagen, Denmark, observed that girls with higher body mass index (BMI) exhibited earlier onset of puberty. However, the trend persisted among normal-weight girls too (13). Accordingly, various coalescing processes have been linked with earlier development in addition to weight and genetics, including, diet, specific endocrine disruptors, gut flora, hormone-laden cosmetics and activity level (14-17). Thus, it has been suggested that the while the environment affects pubertal onset, the timing of puberty may be useful indicator of a girl's physiologic response to her environment.

No known studies have examined the influence of housing quality, or the psychosocial implications of poor housing, on pubertal onset.

Exposures associated with housing impact physiological health (e.g., lead, radon, mold, extreme temperatures), psychological health (e.g., noise, inadequate light), and safety (e.g., falls, fires). Thus, delivery of adequate housing, specifically for children, continues to be a major public health issue in the United States (18).

Presently, over one million Americans are reside in federally subsidized public housing units. The New York City Hosing Authority is the largest public housing agency in the nation and provides homes for over 112,000 children ages 5-18 years. Even so, the agency's buildings are notorious for decrepit conditions, poor ventilation, elevated levels of allergens and pest infestations (19-24). These hazards are not without consequence. The prevalence of asthma among children living in New York City public housing is nearly two times higher than rates of children living in other types of housing in the city. Most recently the agency has been entangled in numerous lawsuits pertaining to inadequate housing quality, including leaks, flooding, mold, warped floors, holes in walls, and broken stoves, toilets, doors, windows, buzzers and mailboxes. Disadvantaged minorities disproportionately shoulder these burdens, and, in the context of poor access to care, face significantly higher rates of morbidity and mortality (18, 25-27).

Predictably, risks factors associated with poor housing determine behavioral health and psychosocial outcomes as well. A 2010 study conducted by the New York University found that students living in public housing in New York City performed substantially worse on standardized math and reading exams than their peers living elsewhere in the city (28).

Adolescents living in public housing reported an increased incidence of substance abuse and gun violence (29). Cumulatively, these risks are only compounded by other psychosocial hazards, and over time become significant barriers to overall health and well being – perpetuating a cycle of disadvantage (Figure 1).

Understanding and addressing housing concerns offer public health practitioners the opportunity to address an essential determinant of health (see Figure 1). This study aims to explore the impact of housing type in a single neighborhood, specifically looking at public and private housing establishments on pubertal outcomes.

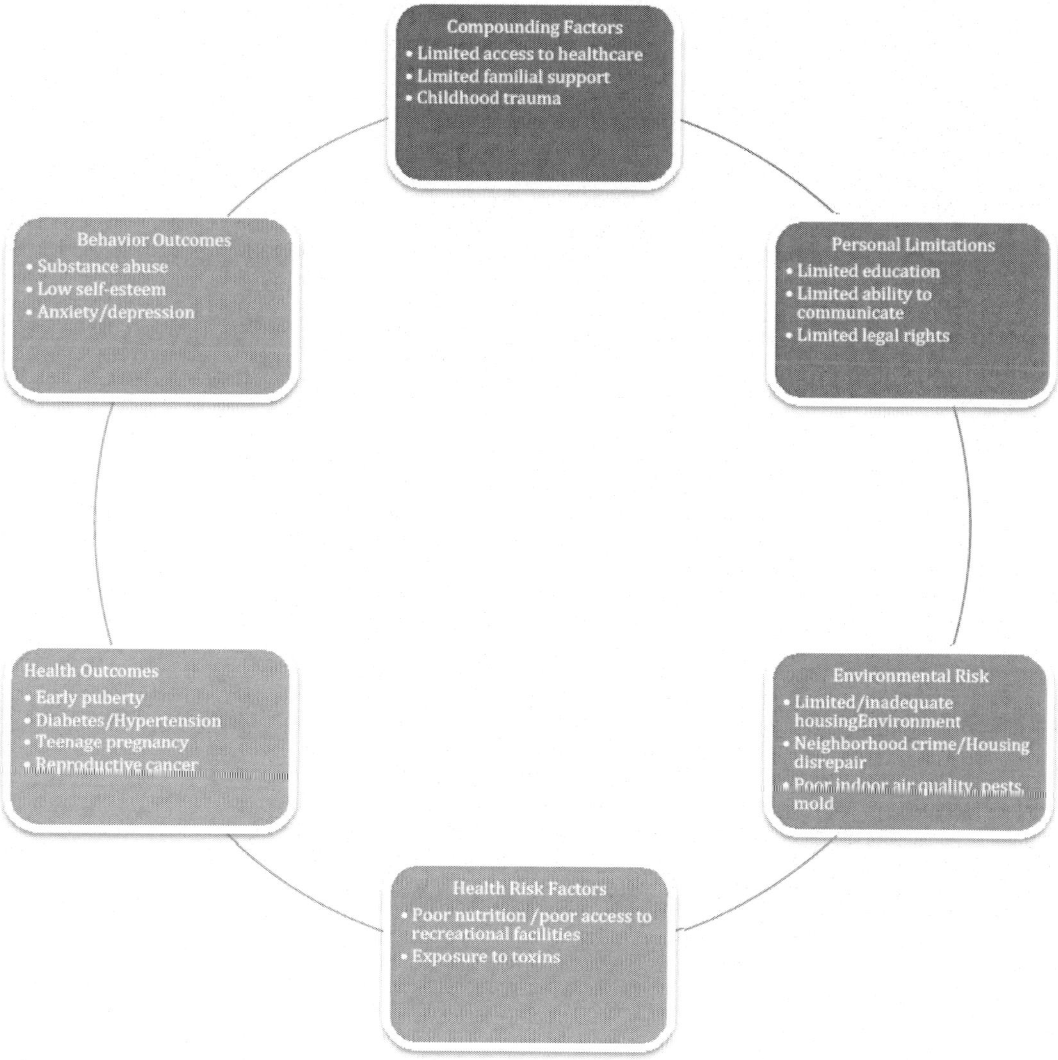
Compounding Factors
• Limited access to healthcare
• Limited familial support
• Childhood trauma
Personal Limitations
• Limited education
• Limited ability to communicate
• Limited legal rights
Environmental Risk
• Limited/inadequate housingEnvironment
• Neighborhood crime/Housing disrepair
• Poor indoor air quality, pests, mold
Health Risk Factors
• Poor nutrition /poor access to recreational facilities
• Exposure to toxins
Health Outcomes
• Early puberty
• Diabetes/Hypertension
• Teenage pregnancy
• Reproductive cancer
Behavior Outcomes
• Substance abuse
• Low self-esteem
• Anxiety/depression

Figure 1. Cycle of disparity.

OUR STUDY

Black and Hispanic New York City girls, ages 6 to 8 years (n = 416), were enrolled in a longitudinal study, Growing up healthy. Comprehensive interviews administered to guardians, collected demographic information, including caregiver education and whether they lived in public or private housing. After 8 years, pre-pubertal baseline information was available for 405 girls. Information for onset of breast development (B2+) was available for 337 girls. Onset of pubic hair development was recorded in 325 girls.

Housing type data was available for 385 girls. BMI percentile information was available for 414 girls. Caregiver education data was available for 397 girls. Caregiver income was available for 364 girls.

Table 1. Demographics of study participants

Characteristic Girls' Ethnicity	**n**	**%**
	405	
African American	163	40
Hispanic	242	60
Family Income	**n**	**%**
	364	
<12,000	59	16
12,000-24,999	134	37
25,000-49,999	114	31
50,000-74,999	36	10
75,000-99,999	14	4
>100,000	7	2
Caregiver Education	**n**	**%**
	397	
<High School	139	35
≥High School	258	65
Girls' Weight	**n**	**Median**
BMI (percentile) at Breast Stage 1	414	76.28
BMI (percentile) at Pubic Hair Stage 1	413	75.28
Girls' Overweight status (BMI>85th percentile for age)	**n**	**%**
	414	
Not overweight	247	60
Overweight	167	40
Age (years)	**n**	**Median**
Baseline (years)	405	7.33

Pubertal onset

Pediatric providers assessed stages of breast and pubic hair development annually. Sexual maturity was established through a standardized method in concordance with Tanner staging (2, 4, 30). Breast development was evaluated through both observation and palpation (2, 4). Onset of breast development was defined as expressing breast stage 2 or greater. We examined pubertal stages (any breast development [stage B2+] vs none, and pubic hair (Stage PH2+), any vs none) in relation to housing, race/ethnicity, BMI and caregiver education.

Body mass index

BMI was calculated from the mean values of height and weight measurements, with weight divided by the square of height. BMI percentile and z score were determined by using the 2000 growth charts from the Centers for Disease Control and Prevention (2, 4).

Ethnicity

Girl's ethnicity was assessed using primary caregiver's report at baseline and was coded as African American or Black; Black-Hispanic; or Hispanic or Latina.

Family income

Caregivers reported annual family income at baseline. Income categories were: <\$12,000; \$12,000-\$25,000; <\$25,000; \$25,000-\$49,999; \$50,000-\$74,999; \$75,000-\$100,000. Income was dichotomized into "lower" (<\$50 K/year) and "higher" (>\$50 k/year) income.

FINDINGS

Forty percent of the cohort was overweight irrespective of housing (see Figure 2). In Figure 3 the age adjusted weight of participants in private housing is shown, while Figure 4 shows age adjusted weight of partcipants residing in public housing. Figure 5 shows the housing distribution for African Americans and Hispanics. Figure 6 shows the median age of recruitment for this study.

The proportion of girls having earlier stage two breast budding or greater, was similar among Black and Hispanic girls regardless of housing type.

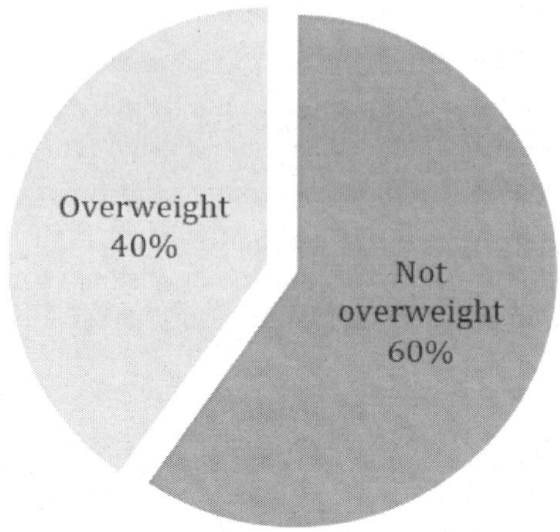

Figure 2. Age adjusted weight of participants.

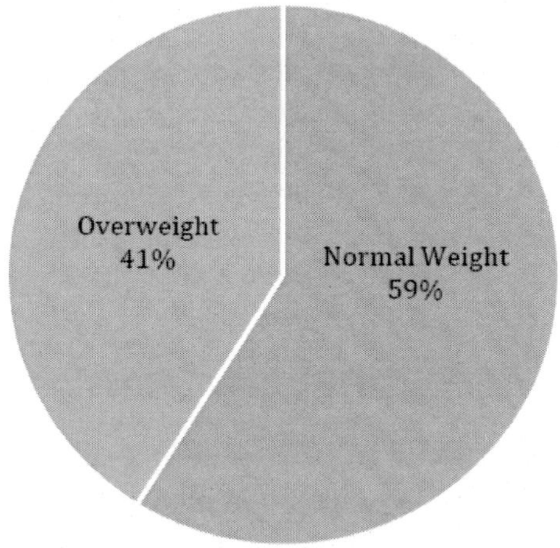

Figure 3. Age adjusted weight of participants in private housing.

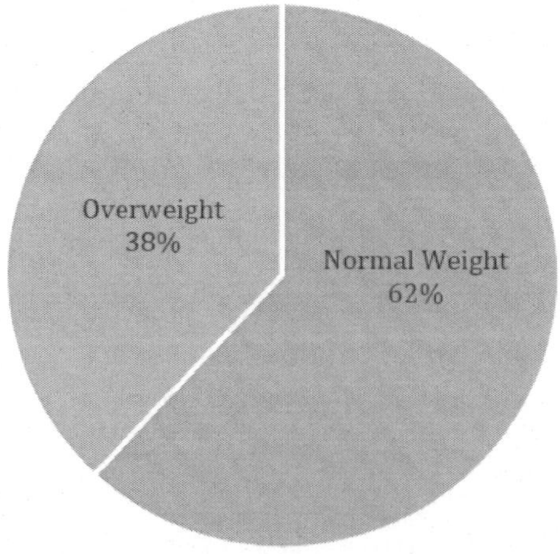

Figure 4. Age adjusted weight of participants in public housing.

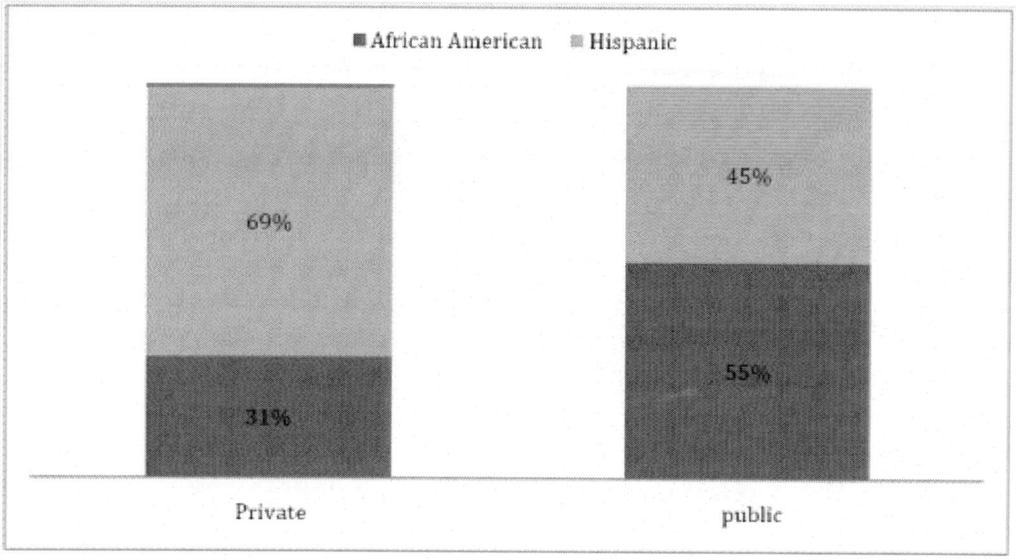

Figure 5. Distribution of housing type by race.

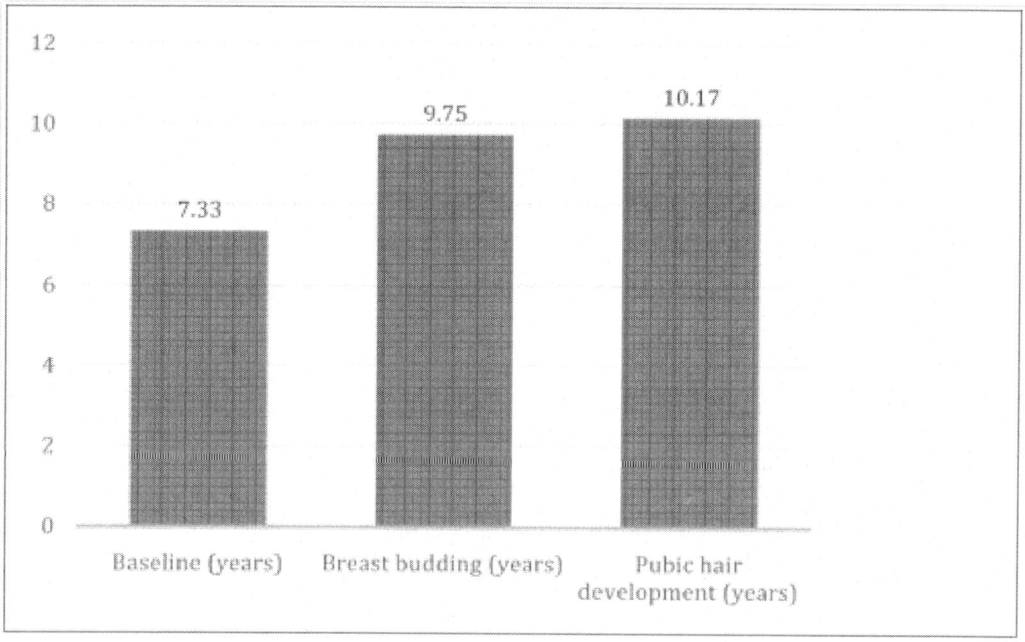

Figure 6. Median age of recruitment.

Pubic hair development occurred earlier in Hispanic girls living in public housing compared to those living in private housing ($p < 0.01$, adjusted for BMI and caregiver education) (see Figure 7). Among Hispanic girls, 48% of those living in private housing began pubic hair development before 10 years old whereas 79% of those living in public housing began pubic hair development before 10 years old.

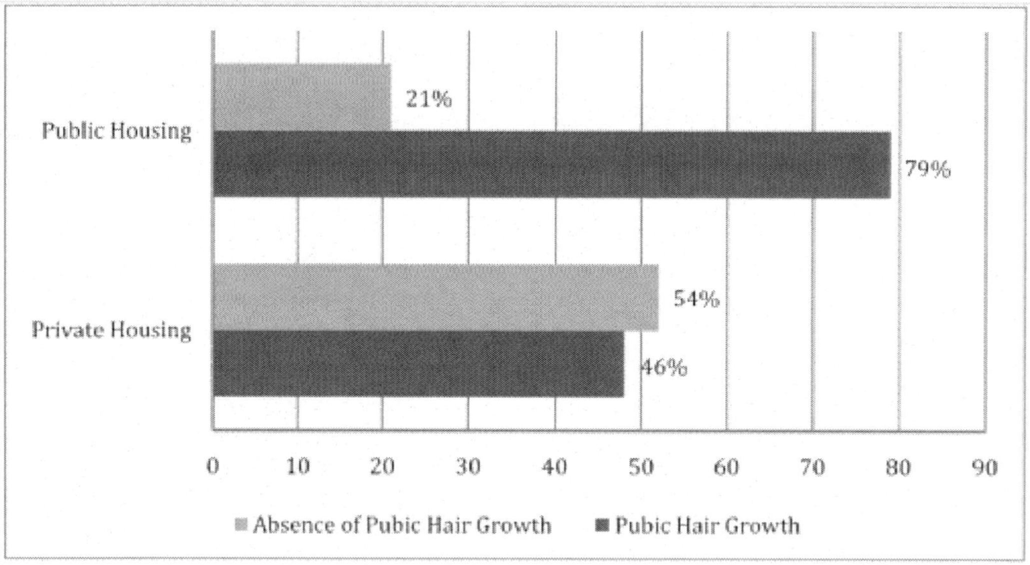

By age 10, 79% of Hispanic girls living in public housing had pubic hair growth. In contrast, only 46% of girls living in private housing had pubic hair growth by age 10 years.

Figure 7. Pubic hair growth in Hispanic girls age <10 years.

Discussion

Intricate neural and hormonal circuits govern the physiological changes that culminate in puberty. New evidence suggests that this is a window of increased vulnerability to environmental influences. Earlier onset of puberty, as indicated by breast development and pubic hair growth, may be an obvious manifestation of the many ongoing internal changes driven by the environment.

Poor quality housing, may alter a girl's pubertal timing via two potential mechanisms: 1) through increased exposure to physical environmental toxins and allergens, that may disrupt endocrine processes, and lead to the premature activation of physiological changes associated with reproductive maturity; 2) through exposure to acute and chronic stress related to the absence of a stable, and supportive home environment, activating hormonal stress responses that induce pubertal onset.

Breast development and pubic hair growth are independent, observable indicators of underlying hormone alterations that characterize puberty. Breast development is primarily governed by the hypothalamic-pituitary-ovarian axis (HPO), and is driven by the pulsatile release of gonadotropic hormones, which ultimately augment estrogen production in the ovaries.

Conversely, pubic hair growth is directed by the hypothalamic-pituitary-adrenal (HPA) axis, and involves many of the same hormones involved in stress response. In fact, children who have suffered adverse childhood events tend to exhibit elevated levels of adrenergic hormones (31, 32) Thus it is reasonable to infer that environmental stress and the resulting cortisol release, produced under stress, may rouse the HPA axis and hasten pubic hair development (11, 33, 34) (see Figure 8). An extension of the stress–exposure disease framework, proposed by Sexton et al. (35), allows us to appreciate the relationships among ethnicity, environmental conditions, and health (see Figure 8).

Hispanic girls living in public housing may be exposed to greater stress, resulting in higher levels of cortisol and other stress related hormones, and culminating in the earlier appearance of pubic hair. However, this is just one of the many conceivable explanations.

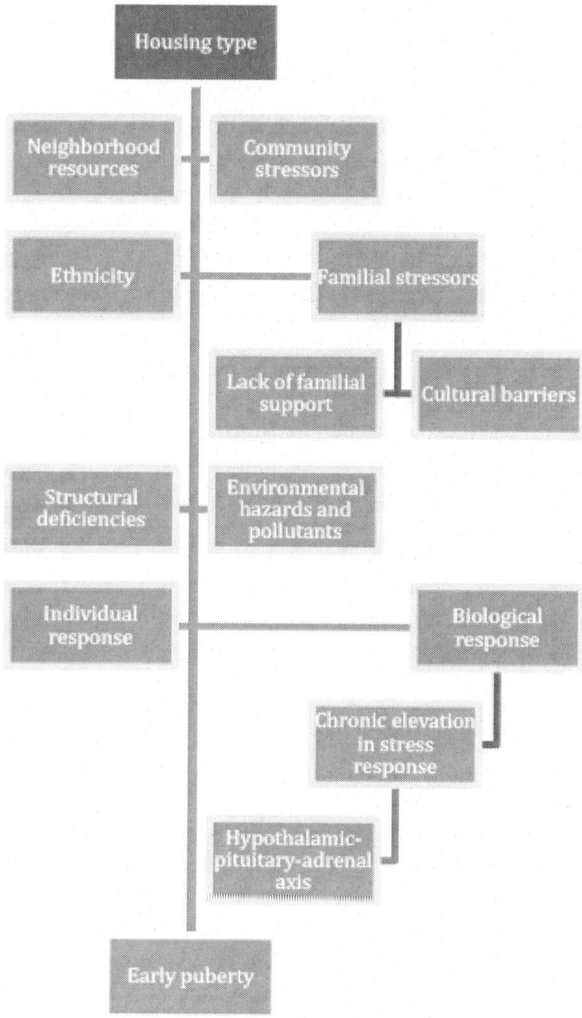

Figure 8. Housing type and early puberty.

Another hypothesis postulates that certain demographic characteristics make some populations more susceptible to particular insults - Hispanic girls in public housing units may be more sensitive to physical and emotional hazards associated with public housing.

Nonetheless, these outcomes reinforce the notion that untimely appearance of pubic hair may be a visible manifestation of a girl's biological response to unfavorable environmental factors. Moreover, these observations may have profound, and somewhat alarming implications as pubic hair growth marks the activation of the adrenal axis.

Premature adrenal stimulation is pathophysiologically associated with several cardiovascular risk and metabolic risks, including insulin resistance and polycystic ovarian syndrome (36-41). Moreover, the chronic stress response and associated pubertal implications may impact mental health as well. Early pubic hair growth is correlated with increased incidence of mood disorders such as anxiety, depression and conduct disorders (42). Undoubtedly, these potential sequelae affect overall health and well being and further magnify existing health disparities.

Fortunately, environmental factors are not predetermined for life and can be influenced by interventions at the level of the individual, family, community and municipality. This includes improving housing structures; eliminating environmental toxins, cultivating community resources, fostering familial support and helping girls cope with psychosocial stressors.

City level interventions include improving structural housing quality. Several studies studying the impact of environmentally friendly renovations to low income housing units - complying with various "green" rating systems - found improvement in overall resident health. Children's non-asthma respiratory problems improved over a one-year interval. Exposures to radon waned, children spent more time outside, and security and ventilation were enhanced (43, 44). Voucher programs, such as "Moving to opportunity," are another approach that has been widely implemented in multiple states. Families formerly living in public housing were assigned housing vouchers by lottery, facilitating moves to neighborhoods with lower poverty rates. Variations of implementations of these schemes have yielded primarily positive results. In children who were under thirteen years of age when their families moved, moving to a lower-poverty neighborhood significantly improved college attendance rates. These children also resided in better neighborhoods themselves as adults and were less likely to become single parents (45).

On the community level, resources that work to empower residents and enable familial cohesion may help mediate the adverse effects of high stress environments. Examples of these include community run gardening projects have enjoyed tremendous success (46-48). From a health provider perspective, pediatricians in at-risk neighborhoods should be trained to routinely screen for social determinants of health during well child visits as recommended by the American Academy of Pediatrics.

Finally, providing training and tools for girls who are chronically exposed to stress may help reduce the risk of long-term outcomes. This involves helping girls develop supportive relationships with family members, especially parents. These may be coordinated via the public housing authorities, community centers or the school system (49-52).

CONCLUSION

This is the first known study to examine the effects of housing type (public vs. private) and onset of puberty. Preliminary analyses point to a possible role for housing type on development of puberty in girls. The study represents initial efforts to explore the relationship between housing type and pubertal maturation.

Our findings indicate that housing quality is one of the factors that may be associated with earlier age of pubic hair growth in Hispanic girls. This supports existing observations that increased prevalence of early puberty among select populations, particularly Blacks and Latinos, is most likely a consequence of social and environmental risk factors, than underlying genetic predilections. Thus, addressing the physical and psychosocial challenges of public housing is a potential area to consider future research.

REFERENCES

[1] Biro FM, Dorn LD. Puberty and adolescent sexuality. Pediatr Ann 2005;34(10):777-84.

[2] Biro FM, Galvez MP, Greenspan LC, Succop PA, Vangeepuram N, Pinney SM, et al. Pubertal assessment method and baseline characteristics in a mixed longitudinal study of girls. Pediatrics 2010;126(3):e583-90.

[3] Biro FM, Greenspan LC, Galvez MP. Puberty in girls of the 21st century. J Pediatr Adolesc Gynecol 2012;25(5):289-94.

[4] Biro FM, Greenspan LC, Galvez MP, Pinney SM, Teitelbaum S, Windham GC, et al. Onset of breast development in a longitudinal cohort. Pediatrics 2013;132(6):1019-27.

[5] Biro FM, Huang B, Crawford PB, Lucky AW, Striegel-Moore R, Barton BA, et al. Pubertal correlates in black and white girls. J Pediatr 2006;148(2):234-40.

[6] Chumlea WC, Schubert CM, Roche AF, Kulin HE, Lee PA, Himes JH, et al. Age at menarche and racial comparisons in US girls. Pediatrics 2003;111(1):110-3.

[7] Sun SS, Schubert CM, Chumlea WC, Roche AF, Kulin HE, Lee PA, et al. National estimates of the timing of sexual maturation and racial differences among US children. Pediatrics 2002;110(5):911-9.

[8] Golub MS, Collman GW, Foster PM, Kimmel CA, Rajpert-De Meyts E, Reiter EO, et al. Public health implications of altered puberty timing. Pediatrics 2008;121(Suppl 3):S218-S30.

[9] Downing J, Bellis MA. Early pubertal onset and its relationship with sexual risk taking, substance use and anti-social behaviour: A preliminary cross-sectional study. BMC Public Health 2009;9(1):446.

[10] Wise J. Puberty timing has profound effect on later health, study finds. BMJ 2015;350:h3318. doi:10.1136/bmj.h3318.

[11] Deardorff J, Fyfe M, Ekwaru JP, Kushi LH, Greenspan LC, Yen IH. Does neighborhood environment influence girls' pubertal onset? Findings from a cohort study. BMC Pediatrics 2012;12(1):27.

[12] Herman-Giddens ME. The enigmatic pursuit of puberty in girls. Pediatrics 2013;132(6):1125-6.

[13] Aksglaede L, Sørensen K, Petersen JH, Skakkebæk NE, Juul A. Recent decline in age at breast development: The Copenhagen Puberty Study. Pediatrics 2009;123(5):e932-e9.

[14] Landrigan P, Garg A, Droller DB. Assessing the effects of endocrine disruptors in the National Children's Study. Environmental Health Perspect 2003;111(13):1678.

[15] Wierson M, Long PJ, Forehand RL. Toward a new understanding of early menarche: the role of environmental stress in pubertal timing. Adolescence 1993;28(112):913.

[16] Bogaert AF. Age at puberty and father absence in a national probability sample. J Adolescence 2005;28(4):541-6.

[17] Kanazawa S. Why father absence might precipitate early menarche: The role of polygyny. Evol Hum Behav 2001;22(5):329-34.

[18] Rauh VA, Landrigan PJ, Claudio L. Housing and health. Ann NY Acad Sci 2008;1136(1):276-88.

[19] Chew GL, Carlton EJ, Kass D, Hernandez M, Clarke B, Tiven J, et al. Determinants of cockroach and mouse exposure and associations with asthma in families and elderly individuals living in New York City public housing. Ann Allergy Asthma Immunol 2006;97(4):502-13.

[20] Rauh VA, Chew GR, Garfinkel RS. Deteriorated housing contributes to high cockroach allergen levels in inner-city households. Environ Health Perspect 2002;110(Suppl 2):323.

[21] Chew GL, Perzanowski MS, Miller RL, Correa JC, Hoepner LA, Jusino CM, et al. Distribution and determinants of mouse allergen exposure in low-income New York City apartments. Environ Health Perspect 2003;111(10):1348.

[22] Peters JL, Levy JI, Rogers CA, Burge HA, Spengler JD. Determinants of allergen concentrations in apartments of asthmatic children living in public housing. J Urban Health 2007;84(2):185-97.

[23] Rosenstreich DL, Eggleston P, Kattan M, Baker D, Slavin RG, Gergen P, et al. The role of cockroach allergy and exposure to cockroach allergen in causing morbidity among inner-city children with asthma. N Engl J Med 1997;336(19):1356-63.

[24] Zota A, Adamkiewicz G, Levy J, Spengler J. Ventilation in public housing: implications for indoor nitrogen dioxide concentrations. Indoor Air 2005;15(6):393-401.

[25] Wing R, Gjelsvik A, Nocera M, McQuaid EL. Association between adverse childhood experiences in the home and pediatric asthma. Ann Allergy Asthma Immunol 2015;114(5):379-84.

[26] Scharte M, Bolte G, Group GS. Increased health risks of children with single mothers: the impact of socio-economic and environmental factors. Eur J Public Health 2013;23(3):469-75.

[27] Newman NC, Ryan PH, Huang B, Beck AF, Sauers HS, Kahn RS. Traffic-related air pollution and asthma hospital readmission in children: a longitudinal cohort study. J Pediatr 2014;164(6):1396-402.e1.

[28] Schwartz AE, McCabe BJ, Ellen IG, Chellman CC. Public schools, public housing: The education of children living in public housing. Urban Aff Rev 2010;46(1):68-89.

[29] Leventhal T, Brooks-Gunn J. The neighborhoods they live in: the effects of neighborhood residence on child and adolescent outcomes. Psychol Bull 2000;126(2):309.

[30] Marshall WA, Tanner JM. Variations in pattern of pubertal changes in girls. Arch Dis Child 1969;44(235):291.

[31] van der Kolk BA. The neurobiology of childhood trauma and abuse. Child Adolesc Psychiatr Clin North Am 2003;12(2):293-317.

[32] Van Voorhees EE, Dennis MF, Calhoun PS, Beckham JC. Association of DHEA, DHEAS, and cortisol with childhood trauma exposure and posttraumatic stress disorder. Int Clin Psychopharmacol 2014;29(1):56.

[33] Ellis BJ, Shirtcliff EA, Boyce WT, Deardorff J, Essex MJ. Quality of early family relationships and the timing and tempo of puberty: effects depend on biological sensitivity to context. Dev Psychopathol 2011;23(01):85-99.

[34] Shirtcliff EA, Dahl RE, Pollak SD. Pubertal development: correspondence between hormonal and physical development. Child Dev 2009;80(2):327-37.

[35] Sexton K, Olden K, Johnson BL. "Environmental justice": the central role of research in establishing a credible scientific foundation for informed decision making. Toxicol Ind Health 1992;9(5):685-727.

[36] Auchus RJ, Rainey WE. Adrenarche–physiology, biochemistry and human disease. Clin Endocrinol 2004;60(3):288-96.

[37] Ibanez L, Valls C, Marcos MV, Ong K, Dunger DB, de Zegher F. Insulin sensitization for girls with precocious pubarche and with risk for polycystic ovary syndrome: effects of prepubertal initiation and postpubertal discontinuation of metformin treatment. J Clin Endocrinol Metabol 2004;89(9):4331-7.

[38] Goran MI, Gower BA. Longitudinal study on pubertal insulin resistance. Diabetes 2001;50(11): 2444-50.

[39] Ibanez L, Potau N, Francois I, de Zegher F. Precocious pubarche, hyperinsulinism, and ovarian hyperandrogenism in girls: relation to reduced fetal growth. J Clin Endocrinol Metabol 1998;83(10):3558-62.

[40] Ten S, Maclaren N. Insulin resistance syndrome in children. J Clin Endocrinol Metabol 2004;89(6):2526-39.

[41] Ibanez L, Ong K, Valls C, Marcos MV, Dunger DB, de Zegher F. Metformin treatment to prevent early puberty in girls with precocious pubarche. J Clin Endocrinol Metabol 2006;91(8):2888-91.

[42] Dorn LD, Hitt SF, Rotenstein D. Biopsychological and cognitive differences in children with premature vs on-time adrenarche. Arch Pediatr Adolesc Medicine 1999;153(2):137-46.

[43] Breysse J, Jacobs DE, Weber W, Dixon S, Kawecki C, Aceti S, et al. Health outcomes and green renovation of affordable housing. Public Health Rep 2011;126(Suppl 1):64.

[44] Jacobs DE, Ahonen E, Dixon SL, Dorevitch S, Breysse J, Smith J, et al. Moving Into Green Healthy Housing. J Public Health Manag Pract 2015;21(4):345-54.

[45] Chetty R, Hendren N, Katz LF. The effects of exposure to better neighborhoods on children: New Evidence from the Moving to Opportunity Experiment. Cambridge, MA: National Bureau of Economic Research, 2015.

[46] Galvez MP, McGovern K, Knuff C, Resnick S, Brenner B, Teitelbaum SL, et al. Associations between neighborhood resources and physical activity in inner-city minority children. Acad Pediatr 2013;13(1):20-6.

[47] Wakefield S, Yeudall F, Taron C, Reynolds J, Skinner A. Growing urban health: Community gardening in South-East Toronto. Health Promot Int 2007;22(2):92-101.

[48] Ferris J, Norman C, Sempik J. People, land and sustainability: Community gardens and the social dimension of sustainable development. Soc Policy Adm 2001;35(5):559-68.

[49] Kohlstadt I, Steeves ETA, Rice K, Gittelsohn J, Summerfield LM, Gadhoke P. Youth peers put the" invent" into NutriBee's online intervention. Nutr J 2015;14:60.

[50] Marshall A, Yarber WL, Sherwood-Laughlin CM, Gray ML, Estell DB. Coping and survival skills: The role school personnel play regarding support for bullied sexual minority-oriented youth. J Sch Health 2015;85(5):334-40.

[51] de Wal Pastoor L. The mediational role of schools in supporting psychosocial transitions among unaccompanied young refugees upon resettlement in Norway. Int J Educ Dev 2015;41:245-54.

[52] Adamshick P. Support for at-risk girls. A school-based mental health nursing initiative. J Holist Nurs 2015:33(3):228-37.

SECTION TWO: PREGNANCY AND OUTCOMES

In: Environmental Health Disparities
Editors: I Leslie Rubin and Joav Merrick

ISBN: 978-1-63484-211-2

Chapter 7

THAI MOTHERS WORKING IN AGRICULTURE: EFFECTS OF HEAVY METAL EXPOSURE ON ENDOCRINE-RELATED HORMONES IN THE NEONATES

Grant A Walter[1], Parinya Panuwet[1], Tippawan Prapamontol[2], Warangkana Naksen[2], P Barry Ryan[1], Anne Riederer[1] and Dana B Barr[1,*]

[1]Emory University Rollins School of Public Health, Environmental Health Department, Atlanta, Georgia, US
[2]Chiang Mai University, Research Institute of Health Sciences, Environment and Health Research Unit Chiang Mai, Thailand

Changes in pubertal timing increase risks for adverse health outcomes. Many environmental toxicants have been shown to modulate onset of puberty. Heavy metals (HMs) have been associated with both delayed and precocious puberty but information is lacking for each HM's mode of action (MOA). The Hypothalamic Pituitary-Gonadal (HPG) axis controls pubertal development through release of LH initiated during fetal development. HMs hypothesized MOA for pubertal delay is modulation of HPG axis' hormone concentration but evidence of this during fetal life is lacking. To examine this hypothesis, we used archived samples collected from 56 mother-infant dyads who participated in the Study of Asian Women and their offSpring's Development and Environmental Exposures (SAWASDEE) cohort in Chiang Mai, Thailand. Maternal and umbilical cord blood metal concentrations were measured using ICP-MS and neonatal urine luteinizing hormone (LH) concentrations were measured using an enzyme immunoassay. Multiple logistic regression analyses were used to evaluate the relationship between maternal HM levels and neonatal LH categories (<0.4 mlU/mL and ≥ 0.4 mlU/mL). None of the metals tested were associated with LH categories although neonate sex was significantly associated with LH category [OR 11.53 (1.12 - 118.94), p = 0.04]. This is the first study to evaluate prenatal HM exposure in relation to infant LH

[*] Corresponding author: Dana Boyd Barr, PhD, Emory University, Rollins School of Public Health, Department of Environmental Health, 1518 Clifton Road, Atlanta, GA, United States. E-mail: dbbarr@emory.edu.

hormone levels. HM exposures in this small pilot cohort do not appear to be related to LH levels.

INTRODUCTION

Onset of puberty involves the development of secondary sexual characteristics, accelerated growth, behavioral changes, and the attainment of reproductive capability. Precocious and delayed pubertal onset increases risk for physiologic and psychological diseases and disorders (1–3). Understanding factors that influence abnormal time of puberty could allow interventions to prevent this occurrence and its potential adverse outcomes. Bodyweight, race, diet and exogenous chemical exposures have been implicated in modulating the onset of puberty (4–7). Studies have linked chemical exposures with bidirectional shifts in timing of puberty (8-12). For example, exposure to polybrominated biphenyls (PBBs), DDT and its degradate/metabolites DDE was associated with earlier age of menarche in girls while lead (Pb) exposure was linked to delayed menarche in girls and Tanner stage progression in boys (8–11). In contrast, exposure to mercury (Hg) has been associated with a decrease in the the age of menses onset (12). Discordant effects between individual HMs suggest different modes of action (MOA) requiring investigation.

Hormones released by the hypothalamic-pituitary-gonadal (HPG) axis dictate the progression of puberty resulting in phenotypic and physiologic changes through adolescence. Regulation of this system is controlled by trophic hormones (i.e., luteinizing Hormone (LH), follicle stimulating hormone (FSH)) and the effector hormones estrodiol (E2) and testosterone (T). Animal models have helped to elucidate individual HM effects on different parts of the HPG axis. For example, Pb and arsenic (As) exposure in animals decreased available concentrations of LH and FSH in blood (13), while Hg and As exposure decreased E2 and T blood concentrations (13, 15, 16). HM effects on hormonal components of the HPG axis in humans are less certain. Gollenberg et al. evaluated the relationship between blood Pb and urine cadmium (Cd) in peri-pubescent girls to their blood LH and Inhibin B concentrations (17). Higher blood Pb levels were inversely associated with inhibin B, and to a lesser extent LH. A stronger inverse association was observed when those in the high Pb exposure category also had high levels of Cd. Collectively, this suggests a metal-mediated hormonal pathway for pubertal delays.

Although HM exposure appears to decrease trophic hormone secretion from the HPG axis, a large challenge in understanding metal exposure effects on the hormones regulating puberty is the dynamic secretion of trophic hormone throughout infancy and adolescence. The HPG develops during the second trimester of fetal life and fluctuates over the course of life. After parturition, a "minipuberty" occurs with a surge of LH and FSH in both sexes within the first six months of life that eventually wanes until onset of puberty (18, 19).

Susceptibility of the fetal HPG axis to HM exposure, specifically Pb exposure, and pubertal onset has been demonstrated in animal models. Delays in vaginal opening and time-to-first diestrus were observed in the pups of female rats exposed to Pb during gestation and weaning (14). All groups dosed with Pb had decreased serum LH and E2 in longitudinally collected samples and the prenatal exposures resulted in delayed puberty. This suggests that the HPG axis may be particularly vulnerable to toxic insults during gestation that could potentially result in adverse outcomes at puberty.

To further understand the potential effects of prenatal HM exposure on pubertal timing, we leveraged an existing Thai birth cohort where multiple biological samples were collected during pregnancy to enable accurate exposure assessment and neonatal urine was also collected. Our goal was to determine if maternal exposure to HM during pregnancy affected the neonatal levels of LH.

OUR STUDY

All study protocols were reviewed and approved by the Institutional Review Board of Emory University and the Ethics Boards of Chiang Mai University and the Thai Ministry of Health. The Study of Asian Women And their offSpring's Development and Environmental Exposures (SAWASDEE) birth cohort is a longitudinal pilot birth cohort of farmworker women and neonates residing in the Chiang Mai Province of northern Thailand. Between March 2011 and February 2012, 59 pregnant women were recruited into the cohort during their first prenatal visit to the antenatal clinic at Fang Hospital in northern Thailand. Inclusion criteria were: aged between 18 to 40 years, Thai identification card permitting hospital and antenatal clinic access, Thai as the primary language spoken at home, residence in their regional district for ?6 months and planned to remain in residence for 1 month after delivery, good general health (i.e., no major medical conditions such as hypertension, diabetes) and consumption of two of fewer alcoholic beverages per day and no illegal drug use. Thai identification cards allowed each pregnant women a minimum of one monthly prenatal visit to an obstetrician/gynecologist. Mothers were followed longitudinally at each prenatal and postnatal visit until three days after delivery. The participation rate was high (59/59 or 100%) but three women were lost to follow-up and one was excluded due to spontaneous abortion (95% retention).

Participants were administered a comprehensive questionnaire at the time of enrollment, at 28 weeks and 36 weeks to capture demographic and other relevant data. Demographic data collected included maternal age and education, household income and occupations. Other relevant information collected included maternal health and lifestyle factors. Infant sex, body weight (BW), body length (BL), gestational age, and head circumference (HC) were extracted from medical records.

Mothers provided blood samples at recruitment, 28 and 36 weeks gestation coinciding with administration of questionnaires. Metal concentrations for neonates were measured in umbilical cord blood samples collected at time of birth. All samples were collected in metal-free tubes and stored at -20°C until analyzed. Neonatal urine samples were collected using urine collection bags during the first week of life and stored at -20°C. Samples were shipped on dry ice from Chiang Mai to Emory University, Rollins School of Public Health in Atlanta for analysis.

HMs were measured in each of the three bloods samples collected. An analytic run consisted of seven unknown blood samples, one water blank and one spiked sample. 1 mL of whole blood and 1 mL of internal standard (250 ug/mL of lutetium and stannum) were added to nitric-acid rinsed polypropylene tubes. Two mL nitric acid were added to each sample which was heated to 95% over the course of an hour. Samples were then cooled to 35°C and 2 mL of H2O2 was added. Once added, samples were heated again to 75°C at which time an additional 1 mL of H2O2 was added. The samples were heated to 95°C and held for 40 min. Samples were cooled to room temperature, 1 mL of 25µg/mL of AuCl3 (in HCO3) was added and then the samples were diluted to 25 mL with 2% HCO3. The samples were analyzed using an Agilent 7700 ICP-MS (Agilent Technologies, Santa Clara, CA, USA) fitted with an ASX-500 Series autosampler. The limit of detection (LOD) for Pb, Cd, Cr, Hg and As were 1.64, 0.13, 1.78, 0.97, and 0.48 ng/mL, respectively.

Measurement of LH in neonate urine was used as a proximal measure of the operation of the HPG axis. LH was measured using a commercially available enzyme immunoassay (Cayman Chemical, Ann Arbor, MI) with an LOD of 0.5 mIU/mL and a linear range extending to 200mIU/mL. Samples (20 µL) were analyzed in duplicate along with blanks, controls and a full set of standards. The 96-well plates were read at 450 nm using a Synergy HT multi-mode reader (BioTek® Instruments) and concentrations were derived using standard Beer-Lambert equations.

Table 1. Demographic and other characteristics of mothers and neonates

Characteristic	**N**	**Mean (± std)**
Mother		
Age (yrs)	56	26.3 ± 4.7
Gestational Age at enrollment (weeks)	56	14.8(±3.1)
Gestational Age at Birth (weeks)	56	38.7(±1.5)
Ethnicity	**N**	%
Thai	11	19.6
Thai Yai	34	60.7
Other	11	19.6
Marital Status		
Living as Married	51	91.1
Married	5	8.9
Education		
None	36	64.3
Some School	19	33.9
Some College	1	1.8
Income*		
<6000 Bahts/month	50	96.2
≥6000 Bahts/month	1	1.9
Neonate	**N**	%
Low Body Weight	29	51.8
Low Body Length	3	5.4
Low Head Circumference	37	66.1
Low LH	9	19.6

* <6000 bahts (~200 USD)/month is considered below poverty level.

HM concentrations were log-transformed prior to analysis. Relevant questionnaire data provided during all three visits were similar so were condensed into one dichotomous observation for each mother. LH concentrations were dichotomized as high (≥ 0.4 mIU/mL) or low (<0.4 mLu/mL) thresholds previously established (17). Birthweight was dichotomized as normal (≥3000 g) or low (<3000 g) based on the WHO international growth charts.

Spearman's correlation analysis was used to evaluate the correlation among multiple maternal HM measurements. Differences in maternal and cord blood were evaluated using a t-test. Logistic regression was used to evaluate the relationship between maternal HM levels and neonatal LH levels adjusting for maternal age, gestational age, birth weight and neonate sex.

FINDINGS

Demographic information from our population is shown in Table 1. Participants were primarily Thai or Thai Yai ethnicities, young (mid 20s), poor, and lived as married with a partner during the study. Over 80% of the cohort had no formal education beyond primary school. The mean gestational age at enrollment was about 15 weeks.

Table 2. Blank-subtracted concentrations of heavy metals in umbilical cord and maternal blood

Metal	Umbilical Cord Blood Geometric Mean	Maternal Blood Geometric Mean	P-value
Pb (μg/dL)	1.78 (±0.15)	2.66 (±0.18)	<0.0001
Cd (ng/mL)	0.11 (±1.70)	0.68 (±1.42)	<0.0001
As (ng/mL)	1.36 (±1.77)	1.80 (±1.62)	0.0017
Hg (ng/mL)	1.70 (±1.99)	1.14 (±1.46)	<0.0001

Table 3. Odds ratio of having lower luteinizing hormone levels signifying delayed pubertal development

Individual HMs and Luteinizing Hormone Associations			
Unadjusted	**Early**	**Late**	**Average**
	OR(95%CI)	**OR(95%CI)**	**OR(95%CI)**
Pb	1.61(0.26, 11.01)	0.69(0.26,1.32)	0.55(0.06,3.72)
Cd	0.527(0.07,3.41)	0.0217(<0.001,0.35)	0.059(0.002, 0.78)
As	0.77(0.07,3.38)	0.42(0.05,1.75)	0.41(0.02,2.47)
Hg	0.85(0.29,2.62)	1.52(.50,5.62)	2.18(0.39,15.62)
Adjusted			
Pb	1.37(0.12,13.75)	0.41(0.05,2.55)	0.65(0.06,4.94)
Cd	0.538(0.046,4.27)	0.016(<0.001,0.36)	0.046(<0.001,0.81)
As	0.93(0.10,4.31)	0.44(0.05,2.28)	0.43(0.02,2.93)
Hg	0.99(0.32,3.18)	1.78(0.58,6.86)	2.52(0.45,19.14)

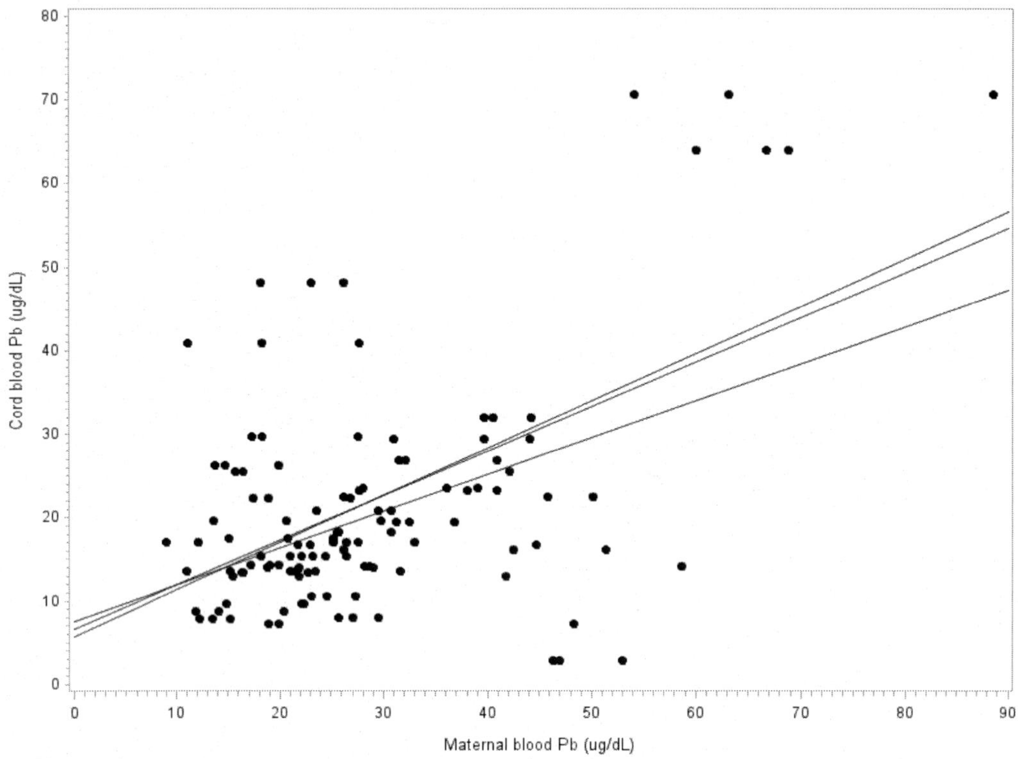

Figure 1. Comparison of maternal and umbilical cord blood lead levels.

Concentrations of HM in umbilical cord and maternal blood are shown in Table 2. With the exception of Hg, umbilical cord blood concentrations were significantly lower than maternal blood concentrations. Hg concentrations in umbilical cord blood were 1.5-fold higher than maternal blood concentrations ($p < 0.0001$). Maternal and umbilical cord lead were highly correlated (see Figure 1) but the other metals had much weaker correlations.

Simple and multiple logistic regressions yielded odds ratios and ß estimates that were not significant for any HM tested. Sex was significantly associated with LH category [OR 11.5 (1.12, 118.96); ß = 1.22; p = 0.04).

DISCUSSION

Our study population was comprised of poorly educated, day laborers working in agriculture who were struggling to live with very little income. The poverty level in Thailand is just 200 USD per month so even if our participants were not considered poor in Thailand, they still are quite impoverished compared to developed countries. Sadly, this is not uncommon in developing countries, and in fact, is likely more representative of developing countries in Southeast Asia. Many of the exposures evaluated, conditions documented, and knowledge of toxic effects of chemicals were secondary concerns to our participants who were just struggling to have shelter and food. It's imperative that researchers focus on easy education and intervention strategies that can help prevent disease in such populations or the cycle of exposures and adverse health outcomes will continue.

To our knowledge, this is only the second study evaluating the association between HM and trophic hormone levels and the first to characterize the association in neonates. We found no significant associations between HM exposure and LH category which is in contrast to a previous report that found a suggestive inverse association between LH and Cd.

Umbilical cord blood can indicate the amount of chemical that can pass through the placental barrier to the fetus. While Pb, As and Hg easily transfer into the fetal bloodstream, Cd is reportedly more sequestered in the placenta (21, 22). This is in keeping with our findings. While the other HM concentrations in umbilical cord were similar to or higher than maternal concentrations, Cd levels were almost an order of magnitude lower. The sequestration of Cd in the placenta may alter functions occurring in the placenta that, in turn, may prevent lowering of LH (23). Despite our negative findings, further study of the link between HM and LH concentrations in concert with additional hormones is warranted.

Despite our extensive HM exposure assessment, our study has many limitations. First, the SAWASDEE pilot cohort was designed for another hypothesis involving pesticides as the exposure and neurodevelopmental deficits as the outcome variable so the samples and questionnaire data are more relevant to these exposure/outcomes. HM concentrations were measured to provide data on potential confounders between pesticide exposure and neonatal neurodevelopment; hormone measurements were added at a later date. A second limitation is the small sample size. This was a pilot, feasibility study so enrollment of additional participants was not possible. Another limitation is that the immunoassay used was developed for serum/plasma and has not been previously validated for use with urine. Finally, this study only represents a snapshot in time of a very dynamic system. Hormone concentrations fluctuate greatly during the course of pregnancy so may still be changing near birth. Regardless, this study provides data to inform future studies evaluating fetal influences of pubertal timing.

Integration into the "Break the cycle" program

The relationship between the surrounding environment and development from gestation through adolescence greatly affects a persons throughout life. The "Break the cycle" program is focused on understanding this relationship and bringing awareness to issues as well as programs aimed to "break the cycle" of health disparity. Our study evaluating the relationship between prenatal HM exposure and neonatal LH concentrations is one step in trying to understand and prevent these health disparities. If we can adequately understand the environmentally-related causes of pubertal timing changes i.e., delayed or precocious puberty, we may be able to develop intervention strategies that mitigate exposures thus preventing the resulting outcome. Figure 2 details the steps of perpetuating disparate health outcomes related to HM exposure. By breaking just one of these linkages, we can improve the health and livelihood of disparate populations such as our poor, farmworker population.

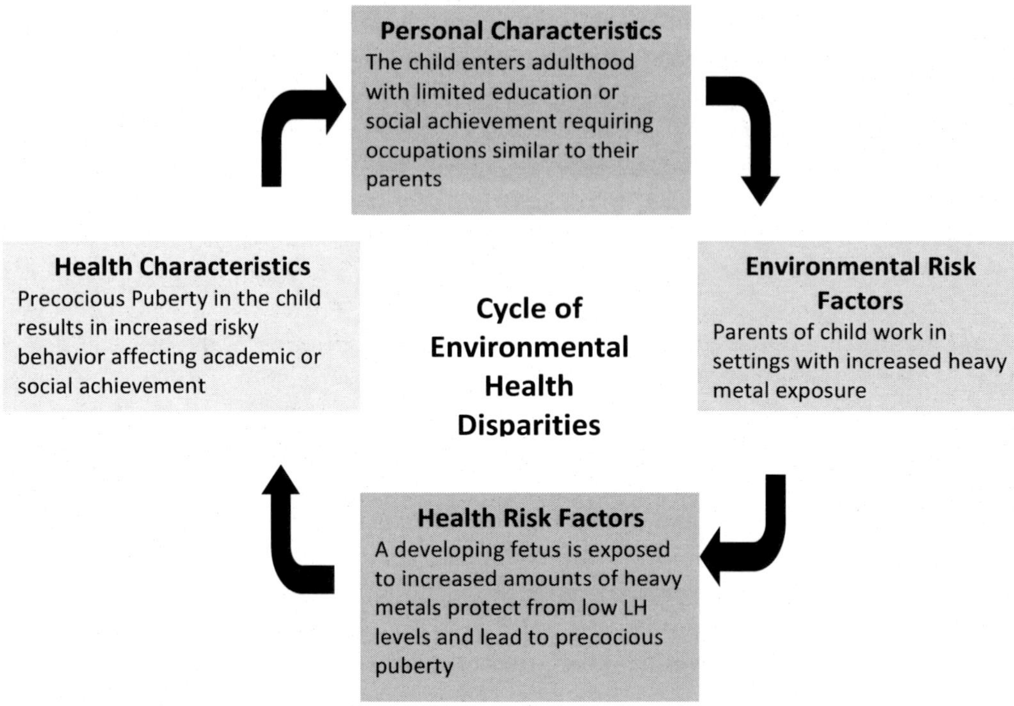

Figure 2. The cycle of environmental health disparities.

ACKNOWLEDGMENTS

We would like to thank Priya Esilda D'Souza MPH and Jordan Cohen MPH for their assistance and instructions with collection and processing of information for this project. We also thank our participants and Chiang Mai University/RIHES staff and team members for their collaboration in their efforts for completion of this study. This study was funded by NIH/NIEHS grants R21 ES015465-01A2 and P30 ES019776, the Thai Royal Golden jubilee PhD program (RGJ 12), and the Thailand Research Fund (reference number PHD/0020/2009).

REFERENCES

[1] Hayatbakhsh MR, Najman JM, McGee TR, Bor W, O'Callaghan MJ. Early pubertal maturation in the prediction of early adult substance use: A prospective study. Addiction 2009; 104(1): 59–66.

[2] Dunbar J, Sheeder J, Lezotte D, Dabelea D, Stevens-Simon C. Age at menarche and first pregnancy among psychosocially at-risk adolescents. Am J Public Health 2008; 98(10):1822–4.

[3] Golub MS, Collman GW, Foster PMD, Kimmel C a, Rajpert-De Meyts E, Reiter EO, et al. Public health implications of altered puberty timing. Pediatrics 2008; 121(Suppl): S218–30.

[4] Mustanski BS, Viken RJ, Kaprio J, Pulkkinen L, Rose RJ. Genetic and environmental influences on pubertal development: longitudinal data from Finnish twins at ages 11 and 14. Dev Psychol 2004; 40(6): 1188–98.

[5] Berkey CS, Gardner JD, Lindsay F, Colditz G. Relation of childhood diet and body size to menarche and adolescent growth in girls. Am J Epidemiol 2000; 152(5): 446–52.

[6] Anderson SE, Dallal GE, Must A. Relative weight and race influence average age at menarche: results from two nationally representative surveys of US girls studied 25 years apart. Pediatrics 2003; 111(4 Pt 1): 844–50.

[7] Buck Louis GM, Gray LE, Marcus M, Ojeda SR, Pescovitz OH, Witchel SF, et al. Environmental factors and puberty timing: expert panel research needs. Pediatrics 2008; 121(Suppl):S192–207.

[8] Blanck HM, Marcus M, Tolbert PE, Rubin C, Henderson AK, Hertzberg VS, et al. Age at menarche and tanner stage in girls exposed in utero and postnatally to polybrominated biphenyl. Epidemiology 2000; 11(6): 641–7.

[9] Selevan SG, Rice DC, Hogan KA, Euling SY, Pfahles-Hutchens A, Bethel J. Blood lead concentration and delayed puberty in girls. N Engl J Med 2003; 348(16): 1527–36.

[10] Williams PL, Sergeyev O, Lee MM, Korrick SA, Burns JS, Humblet O, et al. Blood lead levels and delayed onset of puberty in a longitudinal study of Russian boys. Pediatrics 2010; 125(5): e1088–96.

[11] Ouyang F, Perry MJ, Venners S a, Chen C, Wang B, Yang F, et al. Serum DDT, age at menarche, and abnormal menstrual cycle length. Occup Environ Med 2005; 62(12): 878–84.

[12] Denham M, Schell LM, Deane G, Gallo M V, Ravenscroft J, DeCaprio AP. Relationship of lead, mercury, mirex, dichlorodiphenyldichloroethylene, hexachlorobenzene, and polychlorinated biphenyls to timing of menarche among Akwesasne Mohawk girls. Pediatrics 2005; 115(2): e127–34.

[13] Iavicoli I, Fontana L, Bergamaschi A. The effects of metals as endocrine disruptors. J Toxicol Environ Health B Crit Rev 2009; 12(3): 206–23.

[14] Dearth RK, Hiney JK, Srivastava V, Burdick SB, Bratton GR, Dees W Les. Effects of lead (Pb) exposure during gestation and lactation on female pubertal development in the rat. Reprod Toxicol 2002; 16(4): 343–52.

[15] Davis BJ, Price HC, O'Connor RW, Fernando R, Rowland a S, Morgan DL. Mercury vapor and female reproductive toxicity. Toxicol Sci 2001; 59(2): 291–6.

[16] Sandheinrich MB, Miller KM. Effects of dietary methylmercury on reproductive behavior of fathead minnows (Pimephales promelas). Environ Toxicol Chem 2006; 25(11): 3053–7.

[17] Gollenberg AL, Hediger ML, Lee PA, Himes JH, Buck Louis GM. Association between lead and cadmium and reproductive hormones in peripubertal U.S. Girls. Environ Health Perspect 2010; 118(12): 1782–7.

[18] Kuiri-Hänninen T, Sankilampi U, Dunkel L. Activation of the Hypothalamic-Pituitary-Gonadal Axis in Infancy: Minipuberty. Horm Res Paediatr. 2014; 82(2): 73–80.

[19] Grumbach MM. The neuroendocrinology of human puberty revisited. Horm Res 2002; 57(Suppl 2):2–14.

[20] Prapamontol T, Sutan K, Laoyang S, Hongsibsong S, Lee G, Yano Y, et al. Cross validation of gas chromatography-flame photometric detection and gas chromatography-mass spectrometry methods for measuring dialkylphosphate metabolites of organophosphate pesticides in human urine. Int J Hyg Environ Health 2014; 217(4-5): 554–66.

[21] Sakamoto M, Man Chan H, Domingo JL, Kubota M, Murata K. Changes in body burden of mercury, lead, arsenic, cadmium and selenium in infants during early lactation in comparison with placental transfer. Ecotoxicol Environ Saf 2012; 84: 179–84.

[22] Dietz R, Riget F, Johansen P. Lead, cadmium, mercury and selenium in Greenland marine animals. Sci Total Environ 1996; 186(1-2)67-93.

[23] Stasenko S, Bradford EM, Piasek M, Henson MC, Varnai VM, Jurasovic J, et al. Metals in human placenta: Focus on the effects of cadmium on steroid hormones and leptin. J Appl Toxicol 2010; 30(3): 242–53.

In: Environmental Health Disparities
Editors: I Leslie Rubin and Joav Merrick

ISBN: 978-1-63484-211-2

Chapter 8

PRENATAL ENVIRONMENTAL TOBACCO SMOKE EXPOSURE: HOME ENVIRONMENT AND CHILD BEHAVIOR SEVEN YEARS LATER

Madeleine B Hopson, Amy Margolis, Virginia Rauh and Julie Herbstman *

Department of Environmental Health Sciences,
Columbia University Mailman School of Public Health,
New York, US

The goal of this study was to ascertain whether the effect of prenatal environmental tobacco smoke (ETS) exposure on behavioral symptoms at age 7 years is modified by the quality of the home environment. In a cohort of 417 children enrolled in a longitudinal birth cohort in New York City, prenatal ETS exposure, child behavior and home environment were assessed. Prenatal ETS was measured by questionnaire and blood cotinine. Child Behavior Checklist (CBCL) and Early Childhood HOME Inventory Scale (HOME) were also used. We detected a significant interaction between prenatal ETS exposure and living in a "better" home environment on reported problems in the rule breaking and externalizing domains (p-value for interaction terms: 0.002 and 0.04, respectively), such that there was no significant adverse impact of ETS exposure on behavior among those who experienced a "better" environment. We also detected a significant interaction between prenatal ETS exposure and living in a "worse" home environment on reported problems in the aggressive and externalizing domains (p-value for interaction terms: 0.03 and 0.02, respectively), such that there was a significant adverse effect of ETS exposure on behavior among children who experienced a "worse" environment. Aspects of the HOME environment, both positive and negative, moderated the effects of prenatal ETS exposure on selected behaviors at 7 years of age. This finding suggests that some negative developmental behavioral effects associated with ETS exposure early in life may be modified by the provision of an enriched learning environment as measured by the HOME inventory.

---

* Corresponding author: Julie Herbstman, PhD, Assistant Professor of Environmental Health Sciences, Department of Environmental Health Sciences, Columbia University Mailman School of Public Health, 722 West 168th Street, Room 1217, New York, NY 10032, United States. E-mail: jh2678@cumc.columbia.edu.

INTRODUCTION

The adverse effects of active maternal smoking during pregnancy are well established and can include premature birth, birth defects, and infant death (1). The adverse effects of passive maternal smoking during pregnancy, or prenatal environmental tobacco smoke (ETS) exposure, also have been documented. Most results link prenatal ETS exposure to increased respiratory illness in children, including increased rates of respiratory tract infections and childhood asthma, but reports of effects of prenatal ETS exposure on adverse behavioral and cognitive outcomes are inconsistent (2). Children with serum cotinine levels consistent with ETS exposure had lower reading, math, and block design scores, suggesting cognitive deficits at low levels of exposure (3). Prenatal ETS exposure has also been significantly associated with ADHD diagnosis and ADHD-like behavior (4). An earlier review of 17 studies looking at the effects of prenatal ETS exposure on children found prenatal ETS exposure was associated with subtle changes in neurodevelopment and behavior, but the review noted methodological limitations including confounding factors, imprecise measurement of ETS, and colinearity between pre- and postnatal maternal smoking (5).

Children who experience adverse social conditions, especially those living in low-income urban areas with high minority populations, are at a greater disadvantage for many reasons, including increased risk of exposure to tobacco in these populations (6). Prenatal ETS exposure had a significant effect on child cognitive function at age 24 months, and this effect was greater among children whose mothers reported having greater material hardship, including difficulty affording food, housing, and clothing (6). In the New York City neighborhoods where the participants in this study reside, smoking rates are as high as 27% and 31% to 41% of the residents live below the poverty line (depending on the neighborhood) (7-9). This suggests that children in this population are at high risk of being exposed to prenatal ETS.

A significant part of a child's cognitive and behavioral outcome is determined by the home environment, but finding a standardized way to measure the home environment has been challenging, specifically in nontraditional cultures. One method uses eight subscales to measure the quality of attachment, support, and stimulation that a child is exposed to in the home environment as a meaningful predictor of a child's social and behavioral relationships later in life (10). These subscales include the dimensions of Learning Materials, Language Stimulation, Academic Stimulation, and Modeling. HOME has been significantly correlated with both cognitive development and attachment, in both Caucasian and non-caucasian families (11).

Although the role of the home environment in child development has been well demonstrated, few studies have examined whether the home environment can modify the effects of exposure to neurotoxicants on behavioral and/or cognitive outcomes in children. Growing up in a high quality home environment did not mitigate the adverse effects of prenatal chlorpyrifos exposure (a neurotoxic organophosphate pesticide) on working memory (12). In contrast, rats with prenatal exposure to lead who were raised in an enriched learning environment performed just as well on a spatial learning task as non-exposed rats raised in a similar environment (13). Rats that were exposed to lead prenatally but raised in an isolated environment were unable to complete the spatial learning task, or completed it at a much slower rate (13). Further study is needed to determine the role of the home in moderating the effects of early life exposure to different neurotoxicants.

Because of the high prevalence of children exposed to secondhand smoke in the United States, especially in minority populations, and because many children from low-income, minority, and urban populations tend to have less optimal home environments, this study examined the role of the home environment in moderating the effects of prenatal ETS exposure on child behavior. We hypothesized that children who are exposed to prenatal ETS and also experienced an enriched learning environment during early childhood would demonstrate better behavioral development than those exposed to prenatal ETS who did not experience an enriched learning environment during early childhood. In *post hoc* analyses, we evaluated the hypothesis that the effects of prenatal ETS exposure on child behavior would be exacerbated among children growing up in a depleted home environment.

Table 1. Selected characteristics of study population

	Included (n = 417)		**Not Included (n = 308)**	
	N	**Percent**	**N**	**Percent**
Child's Gender				
Male	193	46.3	158	51.3
Female	224	53. 7	150	48.7
Ethnicity				
Dominican	255	61.1	216	70.1
African American	162	38.8	92	29.9
Mother's Highest Degree				
Some High School or Less	145	34.8	110	37.4
High School Diploma or GED	169	40.5	116	39.5
More than High School	103	24.7	68	23.1
Material Hardship (Couldn't afford food, housing, or electricity)				
No	297	71.2	185	62.3
Yes	120	28.8	112	37.7
Marital Status				
1 Adult Figure	306	73.7	219	72.0
2 Adult Figures	109	26.3	85	28.0
ETS Exposure				
No	279	66.9	182	61.1
Yes	138	33.1	116	38.9
Quality of the Home Environment (total score)				
"worse"	88	21.1	28	23.0
middle	212	50.8	245	79.6
"better"	117	28.1	35	11.4

OUR STUDY

Participants (N = 725) were enrolled between 1998-2006 as part of an ongoing cohort study conducted by Columbia Center for Children's Environmental Health (see Table 1). Participants were inner-city pregnant women between the ages of 18-35 and their children who self-identified as African American or Dominican and who were registered by their 20th week of pregnancy with the Obstetrics and Gynecology prenatal clinics at New York Presbyterian or Harlem Hospital in North Manhattan, New York. Exclusion criteria included women who were actively smoking, had high-risk pregnancies (diabetes, hypertension, HIV infection), or were living outside their designated neighborhood for more than 1 year (14). The study was approved by the Review Board of Columbia University. Children were included in the current study if they had a measurement of prenatal ETS exposure, complete data for child behavior assessed using the Child Behavior Checklist (CBCL) (15) assessed at age 7 and a HOME inventory (16) assessed at age 3 (N = 475). Individuals missing a measure of maternal ADHD symptoms (n = 52) were also excluded, leaving 417 subjects for analysis.

Prenatal ETS exposure was primarily assessed using a set of questions about timing, frequency, and the amount of exposure to cigarette, cigar and pipe smoke in the home. Children of women who self-reported the presence of a smoker in their home during their pregnancy were coded as ETS-exposed and children whose mothers reported that there were no smokers in their homes during their pregnancy were coded as non-ETS exposed. Cotinine, a metabolite of nicotine, was analyzed by the Centers for Disease Control and Prevention (17) in umbilical cord blood and in maternal blood collected by trained hospital staff within two days of delivery. The cotinine measures were used to validate ETS exposure. Participants who self-identified as active smokers were excluded from this analysis, but some pregnant women may still have continued to smoke without disclosing it (18). Children of women with detectable levels of cotinine in either cord or maternal blood were coded as ETS-exposed and children of women with cotinine concentrations above 25 ng/ml were excluded from this analysis because they were likely exposed to active smoking during their gestation (6).

The CBCL is a 112-item questionnaire that was completed by the child's mother at age 7. The mother reports the absence or presence of specified behaviors on a scale of 0-2, where 0 is "not true," 1 is "somewhat or sometimes true," and 2 is "very true or often true." The scores on the questions are grouped into a variety of subscales that measure different behaviors. Prior studies demonstrate an association between prenatal ETS exposure and attention and conduct disorders (4). Therefore, the current study examined the association between prenatal ETS exposure and scores on the Attention, Rule Breaking, Aggressive, and Externalizing problem scales. The Externalizing Problems scale combines of the Rule Breaking and Aggressive behavior scales (19).

The Early Childhood HOME, developed by Caldwell and Bradley, consists of unstructured, 1-hour observational interviews administered in the homes of participants at age 3 years by trained researchers. The inventory is composed of a 55-item checklist divided into 8 subscales. Prior studies demonstrate that Learning Materials, Language Stimulation, and Academic Stimulation and the composite HOME scores are associated with child behaviors (20). Therefore, the current study examined at the relationship between these HOME indicators and prenatal ETS exposure on behavioral outcomes.

Table 2. Main effects of environmental tobacco smoke (ETS) on behavioral outcomes (N = 417)

	Minimally adjusted models[a]		Fully adjusted models[b]	
Outcomes	**IRR**	**p-value**	**IRR**	**p-value**
Attention	1.09	0.40	1.01	0.89
Rule Breaking	1.26	0.05	1.15	0.26
Aggressive	1.06	0.57	1.00	0.98
Externalizing	1.12	0.27	1.05	0.63

[a] Includes a covariate for exact age at assessment.

[b] Includes covariates for maternal education, material hardship, ethnicity, child sex, maternal demoralization at time of assessment, and maternal ADHD symptom score.

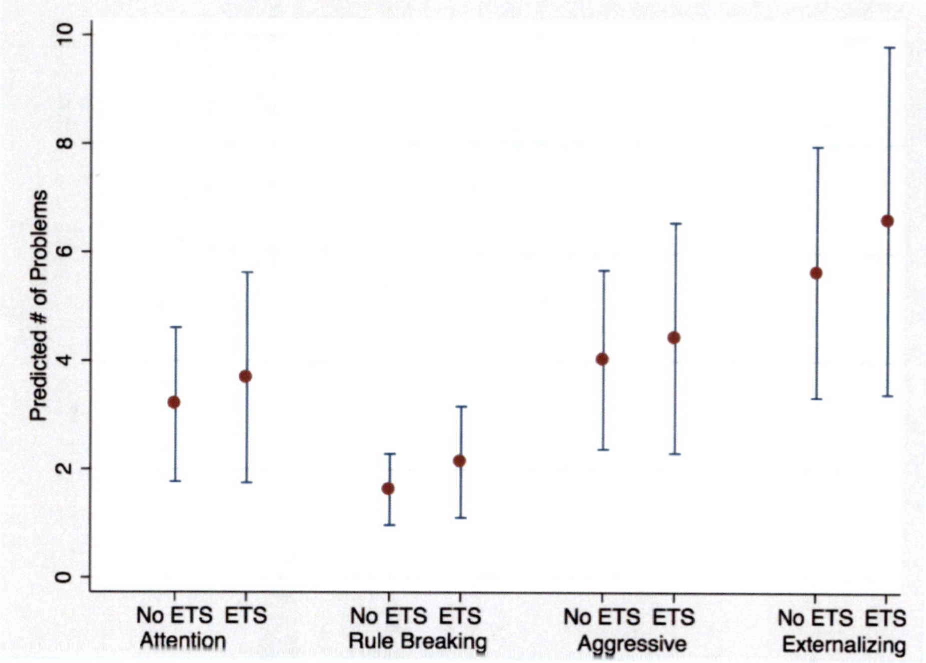

Figure 1. Main effects of environmental tobacco smoke (ETS) on Behavioral Outcomes (adjusted for maternal education, material hardship, ethnicity, sex, maternal demoralization at the time of assessment, and maternal ADHD symptom score).

To find the main effect of prenatal ETS exposure on behavioral effects, we used separate negative binomial regression to model prenatal ETS exposure (present vs. absent) on behavioral outcomes (see Table 2 and Figure 1). Negative binomial models were selected because CBCL scores are count data where the data are over-dispersed (variances much larger than means). These models were then adjusted for hypothesized confounders or variables that improved the precision of the estimates including mother's highest education at the time of delivery (less than high school, high school or GED, more than high school), presence of material hardship (mother couldn't afford either food, a place to stay, or gas/electricity) (21), ethnicity, child sex, child's exact age at CBCL assessment, and maternal ADHD symptoms (assessed using the Conners' Adult ADHD Rating Scales) (22), and maternal demoralization at the time of the CBCL assessment (assessed using the PERI-D) (23).

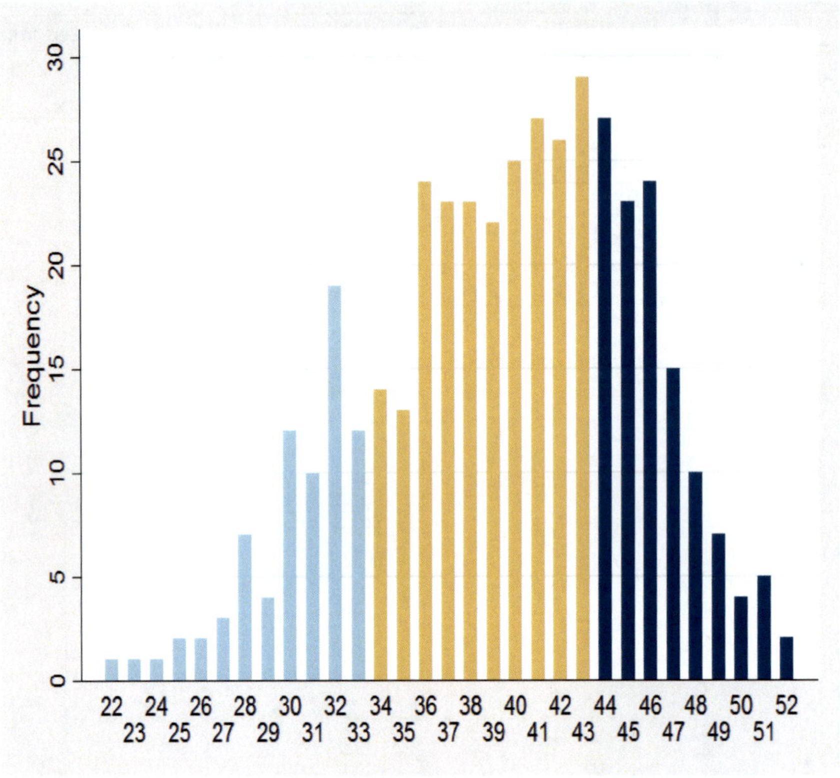

Total HOME scale

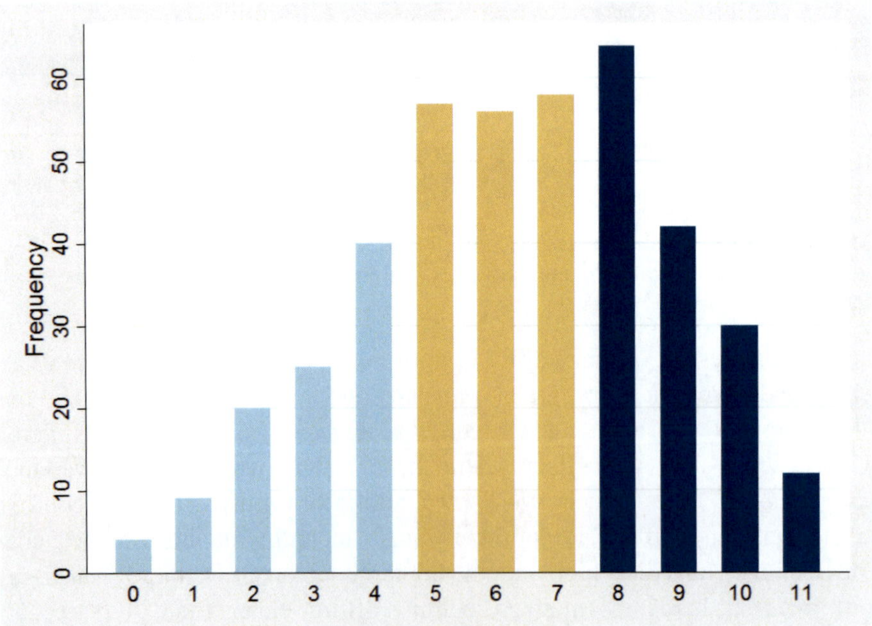

Learning materials

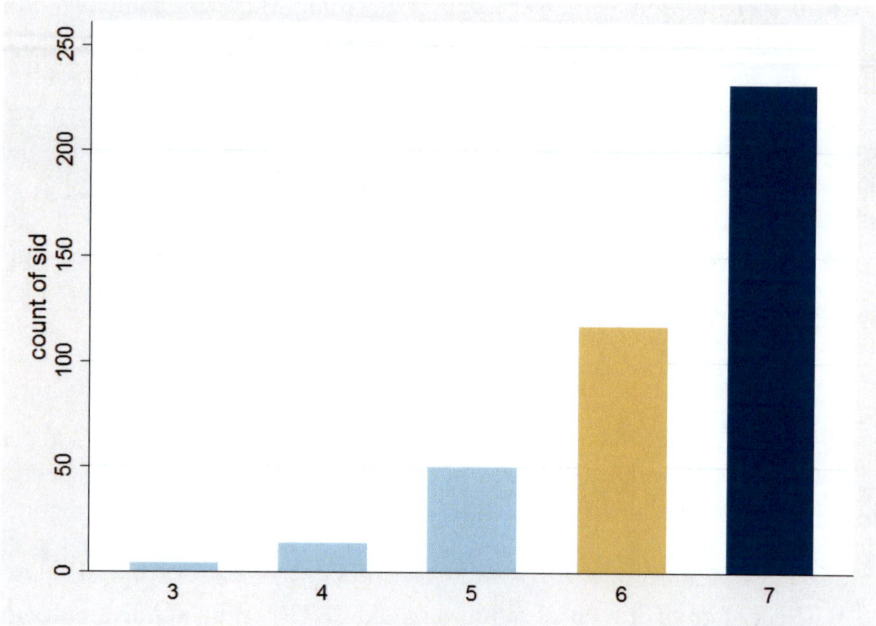

Language stimulation

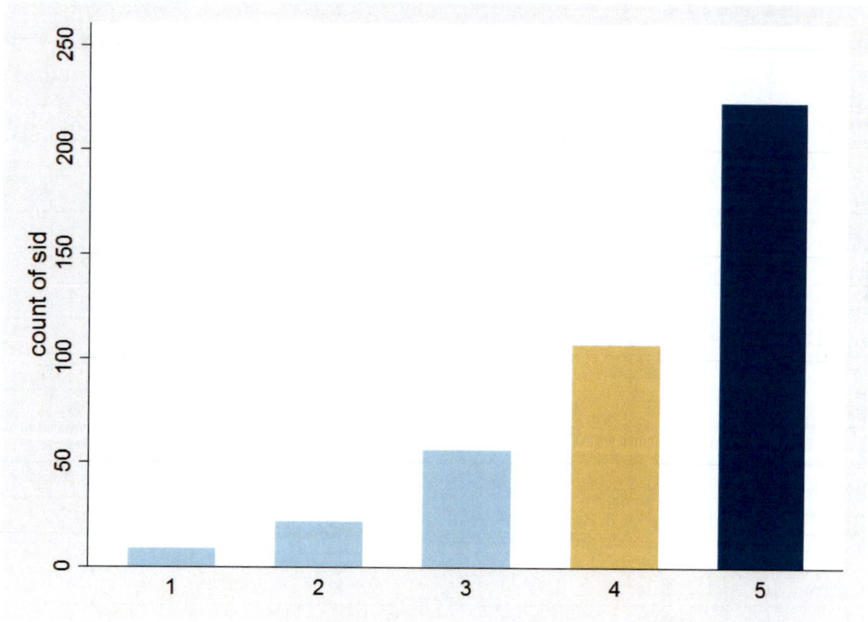

C. Academic stimulation

Figure 2. Distribution of home scale categorization (light blue = "worse"; navy blue = "better"; tan = neither "worse" nor "better").

To assess whether the home environment modified the relationship between prenatal ETS exposure and behavioral outcomes, we dichotomized the HOME score variable using the sample distribution within our cohort. The homes with scores above the 75th percentile were considered the "better" home environment homes, while homes with scores below the 25th percentile were coded as the "worse" home environment homes. We did this separately for the total HOME score as well as the subscales of Learning Materials, Language Stimulation, and Academic Stimulation (see Figure 2). For the subscales of Language and Academic Stimulation, there was no variation in scores above the 50th percentile, therefore, "better" home environment homes included homes above this cut-point. Interaction terms were created for both "better" home (upper 25% vs. lower 75%) x prenatal ETS (present vs. absent) and "worse" home (lower 25% vs. upper 75%) x prenatal ETS (present vs. absent) and added to the prior adjusted models. 95% confidence intervals and p-values were calculated for all models using STATA version 13.0. Results were considered significant at $p < 0.05$.

FINDINGS

The distribution of our final study sample (N = 417) is presented in Table 1. Compared to the full study cohort (N = 725), those included in our analyses were similar to the overall cohort except they were more likely to be African American and less likely to report having a material hardship.

Table 3. Effect of environmental tobacco smoke (ETS) on behavioral outcomes in "better" homes

	"Better" homes		Not "better" homes		Interaction term	
Outcomes	**IRR**	**p-value**	**IRR**	**p-value**	**IRR**	**p-value**
Total HOME Scale: n = 117 (28%) "better"; n = 300 (72%) not "better"						
Attention	0.93	0.73	1.07	0.58	0.87	0.56
Rule Breaking	0.65	0.04	1.38	0.02	0.47	0.002
Aggressive	0.80	0.27	1.09	0.50	0.73	0.19
Externalizing	0.75	0.11	1.18	0.17	0.63	0.04
Learning Material Scale: n = 148 (35%) "better"; n = 269 (65%) not "better"						
Attention	1.05	0.74	0.99	0.93	1.07	0.75
Rule Breaking	0.87	0.48	1.34	0.05	0.65	0.07
Aggressive	0.93	0.67	1.05	0.73	0.89	0.58
Externalizing	0.92	0.61	1.14	0.33	0.81	0.30
Language Stimulation Scale: n = 232 (56%) "better"; n = 185 (44%) not "better"						
Attention	0.92	0.55	1.15	0.35	0.80	0.27
Rule Breaking	0.82	0.21	1.68	0.003	0.49	0.002
Aggressive	0.92	0.56	1.10	0.52	0.83	0.38
Externalizing	0.89	0.41	1.26	0.12	0.71	0.08
Academic Stimulation Scale: n = 223 (54%) "better"; n = 194 (46%) not "better"						
Attention	0.99	0.94	1.07	0.65	0.92	0.70
Rule Breaking	0.98	0.90	1.42	0.02	0.68	0.09
Aggressive	0.93	0.65	1.11	0.48	0.84	0.40
Externalizing	0.96	0.77	1.21	0.18	0.80	0.24

Behavioral effects of a positive home environment

We considered whether growing up in a "better" home environment modified the effects of prenatal ETS exposure on child behavior, as we initially hypothesized (see Table 3). To do this, we ran models with an interaction term between "better" home (upper 25% vs. lower 75%) x prenatal ETS (present vs. absent). We detected a significant interaction between prenatal ETS exposure and living in a "better" home environment on reported problems in the rule breaking and externalizing domains (p-value for interaction terms: 0.002 and 0.04, respectively). In general, we found that among those who grew up in a "better" home environment, the association between prenatal ETS exposure (vs. no exposure) on child behavior was not statistically significant. The association between prenatal ETS exposure on report of Rule Breaking problems was the most different among those with and without more learning materials and language stimulation (p-value for interaction terms: 0.07 and 0.002, respectively).

Table 4. Effect of environmental tobacco smoke (ETS) on behavioral outcomes in "worse" homes

	"Worse" homes		Not "worse" homes		Interaction term	
Outcomes	**IRR**	**p-value**	**IRR**	**p-value**	**IRR**	**p-value**
Total HOME Scale: n = 88 (28%) "worse"; n = 329 (79%) not "worse"						
Attention	1.35	0.14	0.94	0.63	1.43	0.12
Rule Breaking	1.80	0.04	1.02	0.88	1.76	0.06
Aggressive	1.57	0.06	0.89	0.30	1.76	0.03
Externalizing	1.68	0.03	0.93	0.49	1.80	0.02
Learning Material Scale: n = 98 (24%) "worse"; n = 319 (76%) not "worse"						
Attention	1.59	0.01	0.89	0.37	1.78	0.01
Rule Breaking	2.30	0.001	0.91	0.44	2.53	0.001
Aggressive	1.77	0.003	0.83	0.12	2.14	0.001
Externalizing	1.93	0.001	0.86	0.18	2.25	<0.001
Language Stimulation Scale: n = 68 (16%) "worse"; n = 349 (84%) not "worse"						
Attention	1.39	0.20	0.95	0.68	1.46	0.18
Rule Breaking	1.58	0.24	1.07	0.54	1.46	0.36
Aggressive	1.04	0.90	1.00	0.97	1.04	0.90
Externalizing	1.22	0.56	1.02	0.83	1.19	0.62
Academic Stimulation Scale: n = 87 (21%) "worse"; n = 330 (79%) not "worse"						
Attention	1.02	0.91	1.01	0.92	1.01	0.96
Rule Breaking	1.58	0.06	1.08	0.59	1.47	0.16
Aggressive	1.31	0.24	0.95	0.65	1.38	0.21
Externalizing	1.40	0.13	0.99	0.94	1.41	0.16

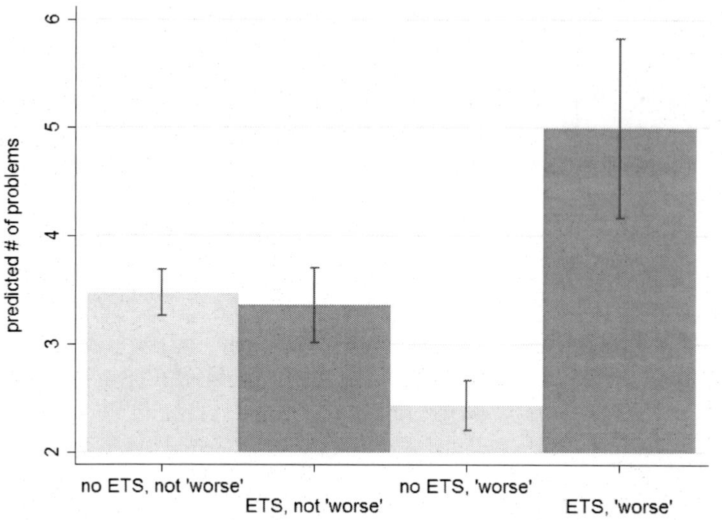

A. Attention problems

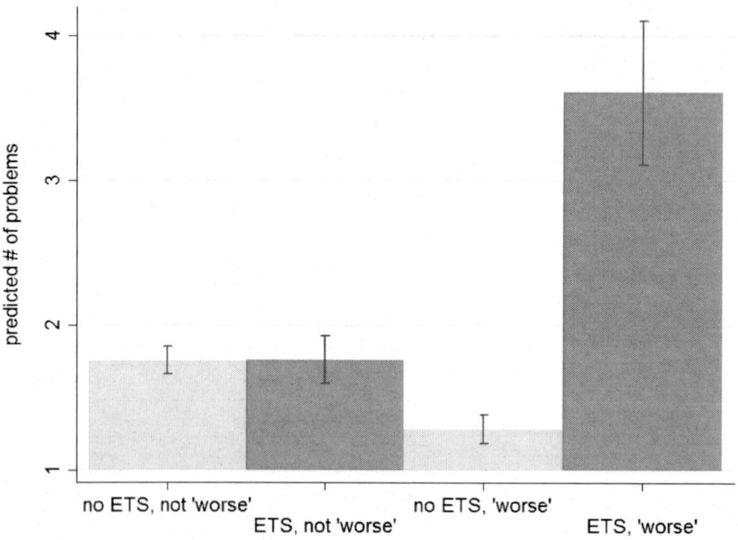

B. Rule breaking problems

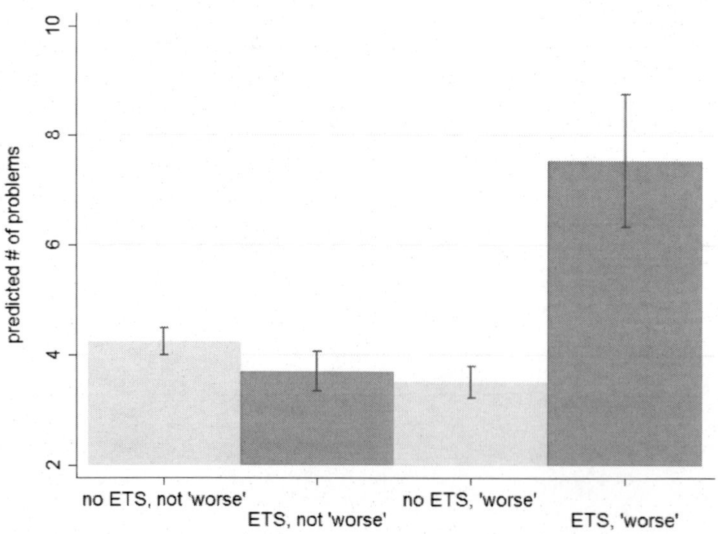

C. Aggressive problems

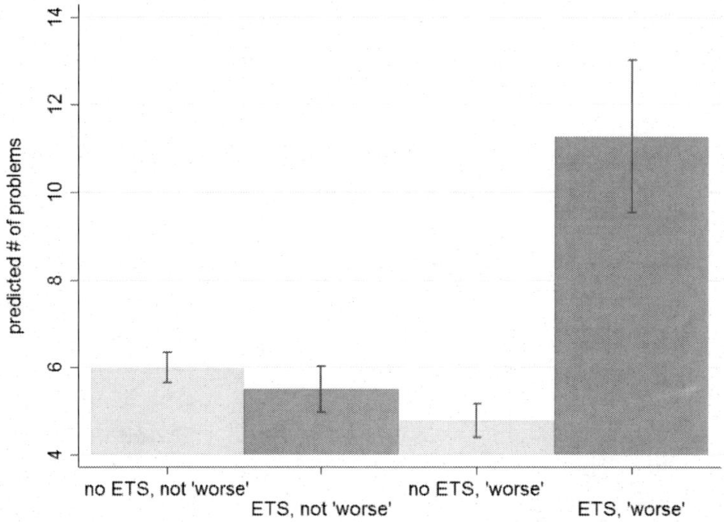

D. Externalizing problems

Figure 3. Association between "worse" learning materials HOME score and child behaviors.

Behavioral effects of a negative home environment

We then considered whether growing up in a "worse" home environment modified the effects of prenatal ETS exposure on child behavior (see Table 4). We hypothesized post hoc that children growing up in "worse" home environments would be more susceptible to the effects of prenatal ETS on child behavior problems. To do this, we ran models with an interaction term between "worse" home (lower 25% vs. upper 75%) x prenatal ETS (present vs. absent). We detected a significant interaction between prenatal ETS exposure and living in a "worse" home environment on reported problems in the aggressive and externalizing domains (p-value for interaction terms: 0.03 and 0.02, respectively). We found that among those experiencing a "worse" home environment (in general), the association between of prenatal ETS exposure (vs. no exposure) on reported number of aggressive and externalizing problems was significantly stronger (see Figure 3). When we evaluated specific domains within the home environment, we found that scoring low on the Learning Materials subscale had the strongest impact on the effects of prenatal ETS on child behavior (p-value for interaction terms for all behavioral domains <0.01). Specifically, we found that among children growing up in homes with fewer learning materials, prenatal ETS exposure was associated with a 59%, 230%, 77%, and 93% increase in the number of attention, rule breaking, aggressive, and externalizing problems, respectively, compared to children without prenatal ETS exposure. Conversely, among children who grew up in homes with at least an adequate number of learning materials, the effect of prenatal ETS on these behavior domains was not significant.

DISCUSSION

In this prospective cohort study of 417 children, we detected non-significant associations between prenatal ETS exposure and problems with externalizing behaviors. The home environment modified this relationship. Children who were exposed to prenatal ETS and grew up in a home with a composite HOME score above the 75th percentile typically had fewer reported externalizing behavior problems than children who were exposed to prenatal ETS and did not grow up in the "better" homes. These differences were small and generally not statistically significant. However, children who were exposed to prenatal ETS and grew up in a home with a composite HOME score below the 25th percentile typically had more reported externalizing behavior problems than children who were exposed to prenatal ETS and did not grow up in the "worse" homes. These differences were fairly large and were statistically significant. This relationship was strongest when looking specifically at the Learning Material subscale of the HOME score.

Learning materials in the home, as defined by the HOME scale, include having toys, puzzles, or games that teach colors and numbers and allow free expression, or having at least 10 books in the child's home that are visible and accessible to the child, or having the family read a magazine or newspaper daily. The effect of prenatal ETS exposure on the child's predicted number of attention, rule breaking, aggressive, and externalizing behavior problems was exacerbated only in homes considered to have fewer learning materials. While our data suggest that the converse is true—that children growing up in homes with an abundance of learning materials have fewer behavioral problems in externalizing domains — these analyses were not statistically significant. This may be due to the fact that the instruments we used to measure behavior and to assess the quality of the home environment are well designed to pick up negative outcomes, but are much less sensitive to positive outcomes. In addition, the cut-points we used to distinguish "better" vs. "worse" home environments were relative to the distribution of the quality of the home environments in our study sample.

We were able to quantify and validate our characterization of ETS exposure using both prospectively assessed self-report via questionnaire administered during pregnancy and using blood cotinine concentrations, which are validated markers of tobacco exposure. Therefore, our exposure assessment was not subject to recall bias. It is possible that women may be unaware of some exposure to ETS, if it occurred outside the home. While blood cotinine concentrations would capture this, because cotinine is only a short-term marker of cigarette exposure, cotinine in blood collected at the time of delivery may not capture secondhand smoke exposure throughout the mother's pregnancy.

While our data suggest that the effect of prenatal ETS exposure on behavioral problems differs by the nature of the home environment, it is also difficult to isolate these associations. Toxic exposures, like ETS, rarely occur in isolation, and behavioral problems can be determined by many different factors, especially when a child experiences adverse social conditions. While we were able to control for many potential confounders, residual confounding cannot be ruled out.

In conclusion, our study suggests that the adverse effect of prenatal ETS exposure on child behavior may be modified by an enriched learning environment (see figure 4). Children who grow up in high poverty areas inherently face negative environmental exposures, including higher exposures to pesticides, heavy metals, and air pollution, and less enriched learning environments as a function of poverty. Therefore, this study could provide an avenue to break that cycle through the provision of an enriched learning environment.

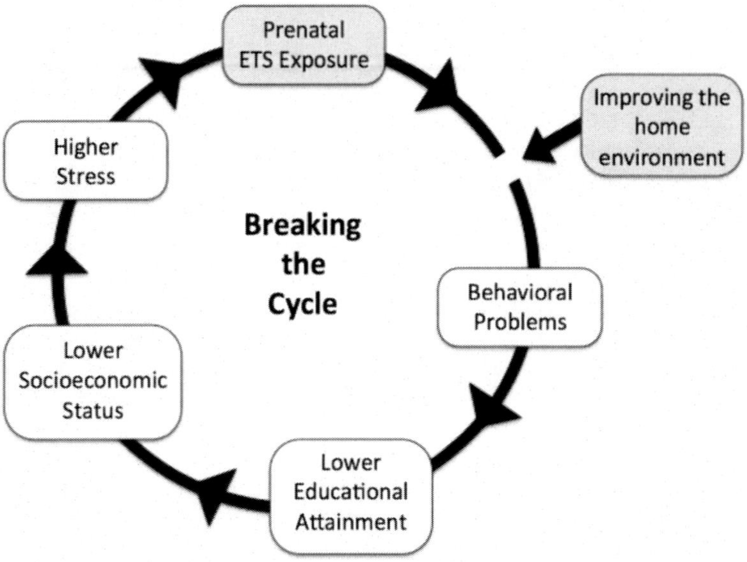

Figure 4. Break the cycle. This simplified cycle shows how prenatal ETS exposure can lead to the development of behavioral issues in children, which can cause children to act out during school and not attain the same level of education as their peers. A lower educational attainment tends to lead to a lower socioeconomic status, which causes life stress that can lead to an increase in smoking behavior in a core family unit, thus exposing the next generation to prenatal tobacco smoke. It would be ideal to prevent prenatal smoke exposure overall, however these results demonstrate that even without preventing prenatal smoke exposure, focusing interventions on improving a child's early home environment may help to break this cycle.

ACKNOWLEDGMENTS

No financial support to declare.

REFERENCES

[1] Smoking during pregnancy. Centers for Disease Control and Prevention 2014. Accessed 2015 May 10. URL: http://www.cdc.gov/tobacco/basic_information/health_effects/pregnancy/.

[2] DiFranza JA, Aligne CA, Weitzman, M. Prenatal and postnatal ETS exposure and childrens health. Pediatrics 2004;113:1007-15.

[3] Yolton K, Dietrich K, Auinger P, Lanphear BP, Hornung R. Exposure to environmental tobacco smoke and cognitive abilities among U.S. children and adolescents. Environ Health Perspect 2005;113:98-103.

[4] Braun JM, Kahn RS, Froehlich T, Auinger P, Lanphear BP. Exposures to environmental toxicants and attention deficit hyperactivity disorder in US children. Environ Health Perspect 2006;114:1904-09.

[5] Eskenazi B, Castorina C. Association of prenatal maternal or postnatal child ETS exposure and neurodevelopmental and behavioral problems in children. Environ Health Perspect 1999;107:991-1000.

[6] Rauh VA, Whyatt RM, Garfinkel R, Andrews H, Hoepner L, Reyes A, et al. Developmental effects of exposure to environmental tobacco smoke and material hardship among inner-city children. Neurotoxicol Teratol 2004;26:373-385.

[7] Community health profiles: East Harlem. New York: New York City Department Health Mental Hygiene, 2006.

[8] Community health profiles: Highbridge and Morrisania. New York: New York City Department Health Mental Hygiene, 2006.

[9] Community health profiles: Inwood and Washington Heights. New York: New York City Department Health Mental Hygiene, 2006.

[10] Bradley RH. Childrens home environments health behavior and intervention efforts. Genet Soc Gen Psychol Monogr 1993;119:437-90.

[11] Totsika VS, Sylva, K. The home observation for measurement of the environment revisited. Child Adolesc Ment Health 2004;9:25-35.

[12] Guilarte TT, Toscano CD, McGlothan JL, Weaver SA. Environmental enrichment reverses cognitive and molecular deficits induced by developmental lead exposure. Ann Neurol 2003;53:50-56.

[13] Horton MK, Kahn LG, Perera F, Barr DB, Rauh V. Does the home environment and the sex of the child modify the adverse effects of prenatal exposure to chlorpyrifos on child working memory? Neurotoxicol Teratol 2012;34:534-41.

[14] Perera FP, Illman SM, Kinney PL, Whyatt RM, Kelvin EA, Shepard P, et al. The challenge of preventing environmentally related disease in young children: community-based research in New York City. Environ Health Perspect 2002;110:197-204.

[15] Achenbach T, Rescorla L. Child behavior checklist for ages 6-18. Burlington, VT:Achenbach system of empirically based assessment (ASEBA), 2001.

[16] Bradley R. The HOME inventory: review and reflections. Adv Child Dev Behav 1994;25:241-88.

[17] Bernert JT, Turner WE, Pirkle JL, Sosnoff CS, Akins JR, Waldrep MK, et al. Development and validation of sensitive method for determination of serum cotinine in smokers and nonsmokers by liquid chromatography/atmospheric pressure ionization tandem mass spectrometry. Clin Chem 1997;43:2281-91.

[18] Lindqvist RL, Lendahls L, Tollbom O, Aberg H, Hakansson A. Smoking during pregnancy; comparison of self-reports and cotinine levels in 496 women. Acta Obstet Gynecol Scand 2002;81:240-4.

[19] Achenbach T, Rescorla L. Manual for the ASEBA school-age forms and profiles. Burlington, VT:University of Vermont, Research Center for Children, Youth and Families, 2001.

[20] Bradley RH, Convyn RF, Burchinal M, McAdoo HP, Coll CG. The home environments of children in the United States part II: relations with behavioral development through age thirteen. Child Dev 2001;72:1868-86.

[21] Mayer SE, Jencks C. Poverty and the distribution of material hardship. J Hum Resour 1989;24:88-114.

[22] Knopik V, Sparrow EP, Madden PA, Bucholz KK, Hudziak JJ, Reich W, et al. Contributions of parental alcoholism, prenatal substance exposure, and genetic transmission to child ADHD risk; a female twin study. Psychol Med 2005; 35:625-35.

[23] Dohrenwend BS, Krasnoff L, Askenasy AR, Dohrenwend BP. Exemplification of a method for scaling life events: the PERI life events scale. J Health Soc Behav 1978;19:205-29.

SECTION THREE: MAKING A DIFFERENCE

In: Environmental Health Disparities
Editors: I Leslie Rubin and Joav Merrick

ISBN: 978-1-63484-211-2

Chapter 9

IN-HOME INTERVENTIONS TO REDUCE PEDIATRIC EXPOSURE TO ASTHMA

Justin Babino*

Center for the Comparative Study on Metropolitan Growth,
Collage of Law, Georgia State University, Atlanta, Georgia, US

Improving substandard housing conditions will reduce pediatric exposure to asthma triggers, which can achieve a broad range of valuable public health objectives. These objectives include: reducing costs to families with asthmatic children, diminishing significant burdens on the health care delivery system, reducing the number of asthmatic attacks, ER visits and hospitalizations, cutting school absences, and lowering the incidence of parents' lost work days. In-home interventions supplement the health care strategies that directly address asthma's symptoms and effects. Implemented in selected cities throughout the country beginning in 2008, the Green and Healthy Homes Initiative (GHHI) introduced a comprehensive program of in-home interventions to integrate lead hazard control and healthy homes with weatherization and energy efficiency improvements. The GHHI attempted to address the health and energy efficiency characteristics of a home through a holistic intervention model, and as a secondary effect reduced asthma triggers in homes. This chapter evaluates GHHI's Atlanta, Georgia in-home intervention services to assess the ways in which this intervention strategy improved health as well as economic and social outcomes for minority low and moderate income families through healthier, more energy efficient and safer homes. Based on interviews we completed concurrent with analysis of the participants' pre and post-intervention experiences, this evaluation of the GHHI program suggests high participant interest, but an indeterminate follow-up concerning the specific issue of the GHHI program's success in eliminating in-home asthma triggers.

* Corresponding author: Justin Babino, BA, 5864 Cobblestone Creek Cir, Mableton, GA 30126, United States. E-mail: justinbabino@hotmail.com.

INTRODUCTION

Among Americans, asthma continues to be a significant public health and economic concern. It is one of the most common chronic diseases affecting American children, the third leading cause of preventable hospitalizations, and one of the chief causes of school absenteeism. In Georgia, there are about 259,000 children living with asthma, and the prevalence of asthma in black children (18.4%) is more than two times higher than in white children (7.8%) (1). Asthma incurs high costs, in terms of the direct cost of care, lost workdays and productivity, and lower quality of life for the individual and the family. However, asthma not only burdens the individual and the family, but is onerous to society as a whole. For example, in 2010 asthma related hospitalizations cost the State of Georgia approximately $200 million (2).

There are myriad factors associated with asthma that may result in exacerbation of asthmatic episodes, leading to unnecessary visits to the emergency department and, in some cases, hospitalization. These include: lack of access to pediatric physicians and specialists, a lack of family education on the best practices for managing childhood asthma, and lower quality of the indoor home environment.

Americans spend 90% of their time indoors, two-thirds of which is spent in the home. Thus, children have extensive exposure to indoor allergens. For children living in substandard or unhealthy housing conditions, this means that their health outcomes are at even greater risk of being affected adversely, because indoor triggers of asthma are typically encountered more often in poor quality housing stock. One study reports that 40% of asthma cases in low income, minority children result from allergens in the home (3).

In-home interventions break the link between unhealthy housing and sick children by reducing or eliminating indoor allergens that trigger asthma. This strategy benefits children, their caretakers, and the community by improving child health and development, boosting school attendance rates and adult work productivity, reducing healthcare costs for society, and decreasing racial and economic health disparities.

The paper examines the Green and Healthy Homes Initiative's in-home intervention program, which aimed in-part at eliminating in-home triggers of asthma. The Atlanta GHHI program did not conduct a comprehensive post-intervention analysis to evaluate the efficacy of its in-home interventions targeted at asthmas triggers. Perhaps this is because the interventions were primarily targeted at reducing lead hazards and not at asthma triggers. According to the GHHI staff person who primarily oversaw the Atlanta program, there were 170 lead hazard reduction implementations and 163 health & safety interventions (4). Nonetheless, using pre and post-intervention interview data that we have collected, our review of GHHI's work helps demonstrate that a relatively modest investment to improve in-home systems and conditions could yield significant benefits for families that are beneficiaries of the interventions and, as result, likely generates significant savings in healthcare costs.

OUR STUDY

This study was undertaken to assess the estimated cost savings to a health care system by employing in-home interventions with an environmental focus aimed at reducing exposure of children with asthma to multiple indoor asthma triggers (allergens and irritants). From the data derived from Atlanta post-intervention reviews, we are trying to ascertain outcomes for children with asthma and their families. In addition, we aim to use information concerning these outcomes to consider potential citywide and statewide effects. We hypothesize that homes in poor state of repair benefit from in-home interventions more than homes in a relatively good state of repair. Furthermore, we posit that in-home interventions will reduce the likelihood of acute exacerbations of asthma, reduce emergency department visits and hospitalizations, reduce school absenteeism, reduce lost work days and productivity, and improve the quality of life for children with asthma and their families as well as provide significant medical cost savings.

This is a pilot study based on GHHI participants' anecdotal reports concerning their experience with in-home interventions aimed at helping eliminate in-home asthma triggers. We did not intend to extract medical reports, count school absences, or verify the participants' statements. Rather, the purpose of the study was to investigate whether participants in the GHHI Atlanta program perceived any benefits in conjunction with their participation in the GHHI program. We sought to understand whether or not those who participated in the program recognized a change in their status, positively or negatively. Initially, a total of 40-50 participants were targeted for this study; however, due to challenges encountered in obtaining participant contact information, we were able to locate only 12 participants, and collect information from 8 of them, through visits to their homes and request for brief interviews. Data were obtained from a survey questionnaire prepared and administered by the researcher with assistance. Institutional review board approval was obtained from Georgia State University for this study. Participants were recruited from internal records of the Green and Healthy Homes Initiative's implementation. Former GHHI participants provided consent for the collection of the information examined in this study.

OUR STUDY DESIGN

In an effort to understand the health and economic benefits of the in-home interventions implemented by GHHI in Atlanta, we sought to build on the body of work that already existed in the measurement of asthma outcomes obtained from the pre and post-intervention surveys administered under GHHI. Therefore, we designed a questionnaire, to be administered in-person or telephonically, based on participants' recall. This questionnaire was modeled after the GHHI post-intervention survey. From the questionnaire, we sought to understand what circumstances, if any, changed in the lives of the participants due to GHHI. The questionnaire also sought to ascertain how the participants perceived their health and well-being before and after GHHI. Further, we asked participants whether they believed the GHHI program made a difference in their lives. For example, we asked the participants to consider, both before and after the GHHI intervention, how many days per month the child missed school because of his or her asthma; how many days per month the child's asthma caused the parent(s)/caretaker(s) to miss part of or a full day of work; and how many times per month was the child's asthma responsible for taking the child to the physician's office, urgent care, emergency department, and/or asthma related hospitalizations. Additionally, the questionnaire was designed to understand who bore the health system's cost for asthma emergency department visits/hospitalizations before and after the GHHI program.

Eligible participants were recruited from a partial set of records of the GHHI Atlanta implementation. We planned to contact the GHHI recipients via telephone or email to set up an initial interaction. However, the available records of the GHHI implementation listed only the physical street address of the recipients, and further information was not able to be obtained from GHHI. As a result, we chose instead to contact potential participants in person and visit twenty-six homes [26] where pediatric asthma was present in an effort to conduct the interviews in-person. Yet, we were able to locate only 12 participants where pediatric asthma was present, and collect information from 8 of them.

Essential to this research project was determining the age, size, and quality of the homes occupied by the GHHI participants. Physical housing characteristics (i.e., number of bedrooms and bathrooms, availability of air conditioning or central air systems, year built, total and assessed value, square footage, etc.) for-forty six of the GHHI homes were obtained through the Fulton County Board of Assessors website. To compare the quality of housing stock occupied by GHHI participants with surrounding housing stock, census tract data describing housing characteristics was obtained by accessing the United States Census Bureau website. We used the data from the pre and post GHHI surveys and the physical characteristics obtained from the Fulton County Board of Assessors website to run an analysis using Microsoft Excel (see Tables 1, 2 and Figure 1).

Census data from 2011 shows that the housing stock information in Atlanta (Atlanta, Sandy Springs, Marietta) is as follows: median year built is 1989; median square footage per unit is 2,200; percentage with central air is 94.2%; housing inventory includes 1,263,200 total units: 58.1% owner-occupied, 29.4% renter-occupied; owner-occupied housing units with 4+ bedrooms is 43%; owner-occupied housing units with 2+ bathrooms is 90% (5). What that census data seems to tell us about our GHHI housing stock is that it is much older than average, much smaller, and generally does not contain the preferred market amenities. For example, many homes have just one bathroom while census data suggests two is standard.

There were a total of 49 addresses (all in Fulton County, Georgia) on the pre and post-survey records. However, there were three addresses for which the researcher was unable to gather information (i.e., physical characteristics) from the Fulton County Tax Assessor's site. According to the GHHI data, the homes that we were unable to get the physical characteristics for were homes that reported having no occupants with asthma. Additionally, for one of the homes that reported having occupants with asthma the record was duplicated in the pre and post GHHI data. In essence, that means that instead of twenty seven households with self-reported asthma, there were actually twenty six out of forty eight homes where asthma was present.

Next, there were two sets of records that had the same street number and name, but different zip codes. For example, 123 ABC St. Atlanta 30310 & 123 ABC St. Atlanta 30315 and 789 XYZ St. Atlanta 30314 & 789 XYZ St. Atlanta 30331. We decided to pull information for the home in the 30315 zip code, which was built in 1952, as opposed to the home located in 30310, which was built in 2007. This particular home reported not having any occupants with household asthma. By selecting the older home, this did not change the median age for homes without asthma; the median age remained 1945. However, by selecting the older home, it did impact the median square footage per unit for homes without asthma.

The home built in 1952 was 1,000 square feet as opposed to the 2007 home that was 2,556 square feet. Selection of the newer home changes the median square footage of homes without asthma to 1,218 square feet; Table 1 reports this figure as 1,161 square feet, which was slightly smaller than the median square footage for homes with asthma. For the next set, we chose the home in zip code 30314, which was built in 1948. The other home in zip code 30331 was built in 1940. This particular home reported having occupants with asthma.

Under the improvement information on the Fulton County Tax Assessor site, to figure out whether there was central air conditioning (A/C) present in the homes, we looked under the heating system and heat columns. We noted that the heating system column either had: "Warm air," "Electric," or "None." The heat column either had: "Central with A/C," "Central," or "Non central." For every address that listed "Central with A/C" or "Central" under the heat column, we marked the home as having central A/C. On the other hand, for every address that concurrently listed "Non Central" under the heat column and "None" under the heating system column, we marked the home as not having central A/C.

Lastly, in order to get a comprehensive assessment of the situation, we contacted the following entities or organizations to access previous data on this area of study: Executive Director of the GHHI and a signatory/funder for the GHHI at the Annie E Casey Foundation; health scientist at the Centers for Disease Control (CDC); and a children's environmental health coordinator and asthma program coordinator at the Environmental Protection Agency (EPA), Region 4.

Table 1. Physical housing characteristics of the GHHI homes

Median (Med) year built	1950
Med year built with asthma	1950
Med year built without asthma	1945
Med total value of all homes	$28,000
Med total value of homes with asthma	$33,000
Med total value of homes without asthma	$21,700
Med assessed value of all homes	$11,200
Med assessed value of homes with asthma	$13,200
Med assessed value of homes without asthma	$8,680
Med sq. footage per unit of all homes	1166
Med sq. footage per unit of homes with asthma	1166
Med sq. footage per unit of homes without asthma	1161
Med # of bedrooms for all homes	3
Med # of bedrooms for homes with asthma	3
Med # of bedrooms for homes without asthma	3
Med # bathrooms for all homes	1
Med # bathrooms for homes with asthma	1
Med # bathrooms for homes without asthma	1
% of all homes with a/c (37/46)	80
% of all homes with a/c and asthma (24/27)	89
% of all homes with a/c without asthma (13/19)	68

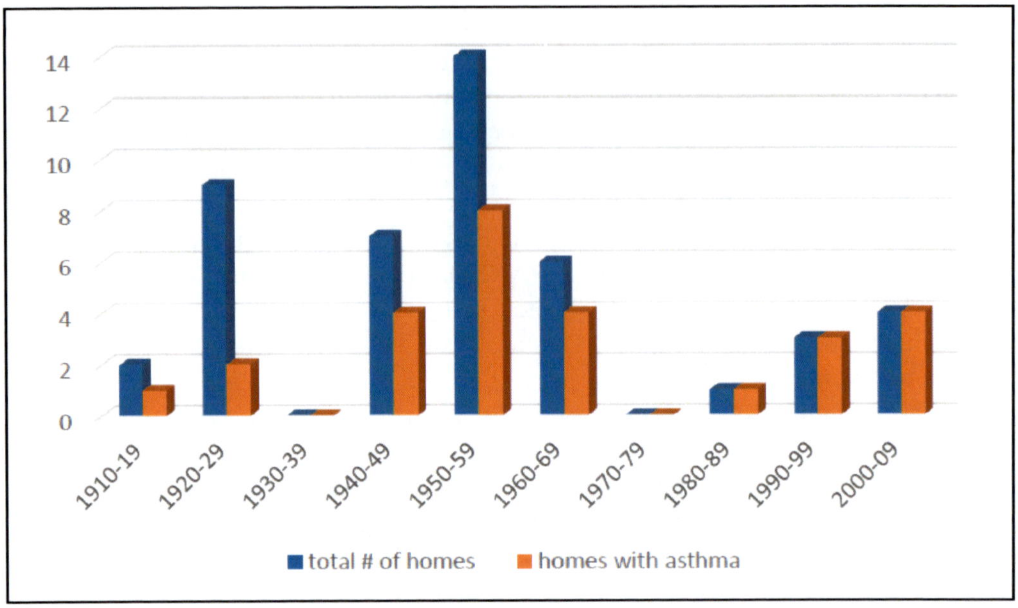

Figure 1. GHHI homes sorted by decade.

FINDINGS

In an effort to identify whether any significant relationship existed between the in-home interventions and the condition of participants' housing stock, we researched information about the age, size and amenities of participants' homes. A significant finding over the study period was that the housing stock information for the GHHI homes program is as follows: median year built is 1950; median square footage per unit is 1,166; percentage with central air is 80.4%; median number of bedrooms was three; median number of bathrooms is 1. Additional data concerning housing characteristics is shown in Table 1.

The data also shows that eleven out of forty-six of the houses (24%) that received in-home interventions were built before 1940. Three out of 27 of houses (11%) built before 1940 had occupants with asthma. The most homes that had occupants with asthma were built between 1950 through 1960, seven out of eight total which were built in year 1950, which is shown in Figure 1.

Results of interviews

We visited 12 out of 26 (46%) of the homes that reported having occupants with asthma. When cross referenced with the GHHI pre-assessment data, the twelve homes visited reported having a total of 18 asthmatic occupants, nine of which were children under the age of 18. However, based on participants' answers to interview questions C-5 and C-6, GHHI Atlanta and Asthma Outcomes Questionnaire in the appendix section, the interviews show that three asthmatic children were unaccounted for (one child each for three different homes). We were not able to get any information or make contact with resident(s) for four of the addresses visited because two individuals declined to participate in the interview; one home had a pit bull tied to the front entrance; and another home was vacant. However, despite the relatively small sample size, based on five interviews we completed concurrent with analysis of the participants' pre and post-intervention experiences, this evaluation of the GHHI program suggests high participant interest, but a likely absence of follow-up concerning the specific issue of the GHHI program's success in eliminating in-home asthma triggers. For example, three of the five (60%) participants informed us that GHHI did not perform a post assessment survey.

Four out of five participants (80%) reported that the GHHI program helped them. Only one participant reported that GHHI did not affect her either positively or negatively. See Question D-8, GHHI Atlanta and Asthma Outcomes Questionnaire in the appendix section. Some of the participants' answers to this question include: "The program helped my family as well as others on my street…especially those that can't afford it." One participant stated, "The initiative helped us…my granddaughter has asthma and I notice the difference when she visits now. She doesn't have any issues." Another participant stated, "I wasn't even aware how much better off we are until you asked me these questions." This participant also stated that she got rid of her carpet and dog as part of her family's asthma management plan prior to the GHHI implementation, because her children would miss one to two days of school per month and adult(s) would miss six partial and fifteen full days of work per month due to the children's asthma. Additionally, she reported that before GHHI, pediatric asthma resulted in taking the children to the physician and/or urgent care two times per month, the emergency department two times per month, and one hospitalization per month. The participant further shared that before GHHI, she spent five to seven hundred dollars for asthma related health care costs. She went on to state that, "Before GHHI, my children were not doing well in school. But after GHHI, my children are doing 'very good' in school, I don't have health care cost, there aren't any more school absences, and no missed days of work."

We learned from the interviews that two of the GHHI participants had to leave their homes for three weeks during the implementation. One participant with one asthmatic child in the home before and after the implementation shared that GHHI installed insulation in November 2012. Another participant with two asthmatic children in the home before and after the implementation shared that in March 2014 GHHI sealed the home, performed lead remediation around the doors and windows, and treated mold in the basement. Both participants stated that the program accommodated their families in a hotel during the implementation. Other participants shared that GHHI's weatherization and energy efficiency improvements included: installation of ceiling fans, air purifiers and dehumidifiers, installation of exterior lighting, sealing of cracks in the home, and remediation of lead inside and outside of the home (e.g., lead paint removal from the porch).

From the information obtained from the interviews, we were able to reconcile some of the GHHI pre and post assessment data, which is reflected in Table 2. After our interviews and adjustments for incorrect, duplicate, and/or incomplete GHHI records, the data derived shows that 26 out of 48 of the homes (54%) prior to the in-home interventions had occupants with asthma. Twenty-three out of 26 of the homes (89%) had children under 18 years of age with asthma. Specifically, during the pre-intervention assessment a total of 59 household occupants reported asthma symptoms, 34 of them children (57.6%). This study does account for homes that reported having more than one child with asthma. The age range for the children extended from 1 to 18 years, the mean age being 7.8 years (median age 6 years).

Other changes noted in the interview data table also shows that in a twelve month period before the interventions, pediatric asthma in 34 children was responsible for: 24 (previously 22) urgent care/physician visits; ten (previously 9) emergency department visits; and 8 hospitalizations. Additionally, in a thirty day period, pediatric asthma for this sample of children caused: 97 or more uses of asthma medication; 19 nights of interrupted sleep; 212 (previously 210) days of missed school; and 41 (previously 20) days of missed work by adults. Sixteen out of 26 homes with asthma (62%) reported that Medicaid bore health system cost for asthma related visits and hospitalizations. No insurance information was reported for the remaining 10 out of 26 homes with asthma (32%).

On the post-assessment data, in a twelve month period after the interventions, pediatric asthma in 34 children was responsible for: Two urgent care/physician visits; no emergency department visits; and no hospitalizations. Additionally, in a thirty day period, pediatric asthma for this sample of children caused: seven uses of asthma medication; three nights of interrupted sleep; no days of missed school; and no days of missed work by adults. Some information in the post-intervention assessment data section is presumed to have stayed the same. However, this does not take into consideration factors such as recipients who might have moved prior to GHHI performing the post-intervention assessment or incomplete data. Our interviews and reconciliation of the GHHI intervention results are set forth in Table 2.

DISCUSSION

The GHHI developed as an opportunity to break the link between unhealthy housing and sick children. The initiative was designed to establish national housing standards and programs that implement a holistic housing approach that combines comprehensive environmental assessments and single stream interventions in the areas of: lead hazard reduction, Healthy Homes, weatherization, and energy efficiency. By blending healthy home dollars with energy efficiency dollars, GHHI is able to achieve a fourfold set of benefits: 1) More efficient use of public dollars; 2) the creation of sustainable green jobs; 3) healthier, more energy efficient homes and 4) better health outcomes for children in terms of reducing asthma, household injury and poisonings (6).

Regarding the rationale for selection, the GHHI staff person who oversaw the Atlanta implementation shared that there was a broad outreach program for the GHHI. This outreach included: educational events, school events, city advertising through MARTA buses and trains, billboards, radio broadcasts, and canvassing of neighborhoods. The majority of the outreach occurred in City of Atlanta Neighborhood Planning Units (NPU's) V, T, and R. Several of these neighborhoods were targeted because they had "ideal" homes, meaning due to the age of the homes it was suspected that they would have lead paint. According to the GHHI staff person, the selection for GHHI was mostly self-selection, meaning the applicants most often applied after viewing advertisement about the program (4).

GHHI staff handed out literature on how to eliminate in-door asthma triggers (4). Additionally, the program's asthma focus was the installation of air purifiers, MIRV 8 filters, mold remediation, carpet removal, and mattress and pillow covers. He explained that asthma interventions cost approximately $500 per home and require relatively low-level skills (4).

Table 2. Relation to asthma

	# of homes w/asthma occupants	# of homes w/children under 18 w/asthma	# of children with asthma	Avg. Age	# of UC/clinic visits	# of ER visits	# of asthma related hospitalizations	# of times rescue inhaler or nebulizer used	# of nights that child was up in the middle of the night	# of missed days of school/ daycare	# of total days of work missed by adult(s)	Who bore health system cost for asthma ER visits/hospitalizations
Pre-Intervention Asthma Assessment	26	23	34	7.8	24	10	8	97+	19	212	41	16 Medicaid 10 not reported
Post-Intervention A Asthma Assessment	26	23	34	7.8	2	0	0	7	3	0	0	

Participants had to submit required documentation to prove that they owned the home. If they rented, then they had to submit documentation from the landlord that he/she owned the property. Furthermore, participants had to submit proof that children lived in the home. Additionally, participants had to submit income statements and, if they did not work, then proof of unemployment was required.

Notably, asthma was not a requirement for eligibility to participate in the program. Also, we learned from an interview with a GHHI staff member that filling out the pre or post-assessment survey was not required (4). Perhaps this explains why the sub-set of data we received from GHHI was incomplete. According to the GHHI staff person who oversaw implementation of the Atlanta in-home interventions, the relatively low yield of data resulted from the fact that he had difficulty contacting the recipients (e.g., recipients would not return GHHI's calls, they had moved, etc.) (4).

The data listed in Table 1 shows that the homes with asthma are marginally newer and larger. Our hypothesis that homes in poor state of repair benefit from in-home interventions more than homes in a relatively good state of repair could not be validated because of an unsubstantiated correlation between the age and size of the GHHI housing stock and the state of repair. We were unable to find out whether there is a presumptive rule of thumb that suggest houses of a certain size (i.e., 1200 sq. ft. or less) or age (i.e., 50 years or older) are "substandard" (due to size, presence of lead paint, asbestos, etc.). However, there is literature that suggest that unsafe and unhealthy housing (i.e., those marked with elevated levels of dust mites, mice allergens, mold spores, water damage, inadequate insulation and air leakage) results in housing-based illness like asthma (5, 6).

Furthermore, the data in Table 1 shows that the homes with asthma had a higher total and assessed value than the homes without asthma. Also, the percentage of homes with asthma and A/C is higher than the percentage of homes without asthma and A/C. We noted that for air circulation, the homes visited relied on air conditioning (non-central or central), open windows, and electric fans. Although the homes without A/C have a lower incidence of pediatric asthma, perhaps this so because they rely on open windows for air circulation. Older homes that rely on A/C may circulate asthma triggers throughout the system, hence retaining and exacerbating in-door allergens and irritants.

However, a possible limitation regarding the home circulation is that just because a home reports "Central" heat may not mean that there is also central air conditioning. This became obvious when we were doing field interviews and noted that one of the homes listed as having central A/C, based on Fulton County Tax Assessor information, in fact had a few window air conditioning units. Thus, the percentage of GHHI homes with central A/C may be overstated. Further, because we were not able to visit every address in the data set to confirm whether they had central A/C, the data analysis is limited with respect to knowing for sure this particular physical characteristic of the properties.

While this analysis sought to evaluate the cost benefit of GHHI's Atlanta, Georgia in-home intervention services, it is important to note that the information reported is limited. Although the data listed in Table 2 shows dramatic changes, we were not able to calculate the estimated cost of the interventions versus the major benefit to the health for minority low and moderate income families and to the cost savings of the health care delivery system. Unfortunately, we were not able to interview all 26 homes that reported having children with asthma and we have no way of knowing for sure how accurate and reliable the pre and post GHHI records are. For example, the post-assessment records reported that one home had one asthmatic child living in the home after the implementation, but the participant stated there were two. Another home was reported as having no children under 18 years of age with asthma and there was one. Moreover, two of the homes that participated in the GHHI pre-assessment were not accounted for in the GHHI post-assessment due to relocation and death. However, we inadvertently visited the homeowner that GHHI reported as deceased and learned that the homeowner was not deceased, but had lived there for nineteen years and recalled the GHHI implementation. We also visited the home GHHI reported as a relocation and this home was vacant.

This study is limited by the retrospective nature of the data and by the method of data collection and limited GHHI Atlanta data. Specifically, limitations regarding the interviews included: a couple of participants indicated that another family member (i.e., primary caretaker would have more information regarding the number of missed days of school, cost of healthcare, etc.); recipients who promised to conduct telephone interviews did not return the researcher's calls; and recipients did not have time to participate in the interview. Furthermore, the study is limited by lack of response to emails and phone calls made to GHHI professionals, which presented a significant barrier to securing federal summary data for the GHHI program. Lastly, this research is limited by constraints of time.

Despite the limitations, this study has important implications for leveraging public and private resources to support comprehensive initiatives like GHHI, which can ultimately yield health care cost savings as well as break the link between unhealthy housing and sick children. There is literature that supports our hypothesis that in-home interventions will provide medical cost savings, reduced school absenteeism, reduced lost work days and productivity, and improved quality of life for children with asthma and their families (6-9).

A 1997 Atlanta program, known as ZAP Asthma, was a 16 member public, private partnership created to reduce preventable morbidity and mortality from asthma for children living in Atlanta's Empowerment Zone (34 of Atlanta's poorest neighborhoods). Utilizing an "action research/participatory research model," known asthma triggers in the home environment of study participants were identified and ameliorated, utilizing the skills of trained community health workers, who assisted families in sustaining the in-home interventions. The study monitored the impact of reductions in exposure to cockroach antigens, dust mites, and environmental tobacco smoke on the severity of the disease, and, on cost of care, schools days missed, and parent work days missed. Despite funding obstacles, ZAP concluded in-home interventions provided medical cost savings, reduced school absenteeism, reduced lost work days and productivity, and improved quality of life for children with asthma and their families (7).

Next, a mayoral newspaper reports that using the GHHI approach, cities can: improve school performance and attendance and reduce health care costs caused by reductions in asthma episodes (6). The same report also noted that the first 180 homes in the initial GHHI Pilot Project in Baltimore evidenced cost savings in some homes over 25% (6). In effect, the money invested in interventions in the home for one case study paid for itself by avoided health care cost from the asthmatic child not having to be repeatedly hospitalized for asthma episodes.

Another example that helps children and their families manage asthma more effectively and saves the healthcare system money is the Community Asthma Initiative (CAI) based in Boston, Massachusetts. CAI uses community health workers to visit families of children with serious asthma, in an effort to help them understand what can trigger attacks and how to avoid them. The CAI even pays for equipment such as vacuum cleaners and pest management supplies to help reduce indoor environmental pollutants that exacerbate asthma symptoms (8). Researchers who performed a cost analysis for the CAI reported that these programs work. The CAI saved more than $80,000 in the first three years of the program and demonstrated a return on investment (ROI) of 1.33. The initiative also contributed to reductions in ED visits (57 percent) and hospital admissions (80 percent), and fewer reported school and work absences (8, 9).

In-home interventions provide significant opportunities to break the link between unhealthy housing and sick children. However, comprehensive initiatives like GHHI must account for other factors that contribute to in home asthma triggers. For example, we observed that two of the participants smoked cigarettes, and another participant had a dog; two of these homes had children with asthma. Additionally, we observed that one home that was elevated on bricks was near train tracks (MARTA and freight rails), a tire depot, and next to several of abandoned homes. Because the link between the environment and asthma is complicated by other factors including tobacco smoke and environmental pollution, in-home interventions is only one component of a multifaceted approach to decreasing asthma prevalence.

CONCLUSION

This paper has focused narrowly on a population of 26 homes in several of Atlanta's low and moderate income, predominantly African American neighborhoods. The paper underscores the importance of an in-home intervention program (such as the GHHI program studied in detail here) as one, low-cost, way to create more healthy living environments for some of our most vulnerable children – asthmatic children from low-income minority families. This report also highlights the much broader policy implication for cities across the country, such as Atlanta, that have a significant population of older, smaller, substandard housing stock. The serious deficiencies of older housing stock and the acute vulnerability of asthmatic children are destined to continue to be a costly combination for tens of thousands of asthmatic minority children for decades to come. It is critical that federal, state, and local governments consider how to fund in-home intervention programs, because the economics of building construction and the housing industry do not favor developers replacing these older homes short of massive shifts at the neighborhood level in a city's residential real estate market. The age and condition of this urban housing stock forces average home values so low that developers are, at a minimum, hard-pressed from an economic standpoint to develop new homes in such low-cost markets that would include amenities and features that would help fight asthma triggers. In short, the problem of older housing stock exacerbating pediatric asthma is likely an issue of long-term concern. It is, therefore, critical to continue efforts to identify and implement the most effective and cost-efficient in-home interventions to eliminate asthma triggers.

ACKNOWLEDGMENTS

Funding for development of this study was provided, in part, by the Southeast Pediatric Environmental Health Specialty Unit at Emory University.

The author would like to acknowledge John T. Marshall, assistant professor of law at Georgia State University College of Law in Atlanta. His guidance, wisdom, and valuable comments contributed tremendously to the completion of this project.

Additionally, the author wishes to express his gratitude to Lauline Babino for her unwavering support and encouragement, which also contributed to the completion of this project.

APPENDIX

GHHI Atlanta and Asthma Outcomes Questionnaire

Section A. *Introduction*

Omitted.

Section B. *Consent to Conduct Questionnaire*

Omitted.

Section C. *Asthma History Pre-GHHI Intervention*

C-1. How many people, including you, lived in your home?

C-2. How many were children?

C-3. Did any household occupants, of any age, have asthma?

○ Yes ○ No

C-4. If yes, how many?

C-5. Do any children under the age of 18 have asthma?

○ Yes ○ No

C-6. How many of those children under the age of 18 suffered from asthma?

C-7. Before the GHHI program entered your home to make its changes, did the children living at home miss school/daycare because of their asthma?

○ Yes ○ No

C-8. If yes, approximately how many days per month was asthma responsible for their missing school?

C-9. If yes, approximately how many days per month the child's/children's asthma cause adult(s) in the household to miss part of a day of work?

C-10. If yes, approximately how many times per month was asthma responsible for your taking the child/children to:

the clinic and/or urgent care

the emergency room department

asthma related hospitalizations

C-11. How much money did you spend per month on asthma urgent care/ER visits/hospitalizations before the GHHI program??

C-12. Who bore health system cost for asthma ER visits/hospitalizations before the GHHI program?

◯ Medicaid ◯ Medicare ◯ Private Insurance ◯ Hospital ◯ Self

C-13. Before the GHHI program entered your home to make its changes, how were the child/children doing in school?

◯ not well ◯ well ◯ good ◯ very good

Did the same number of people live in your home after the GHHI program began?
◯ Yes ◯ No

How many were children?

How many of those children suffered from asthma?

Section D: *Asthma History Post GHHI Intervention*

D-1. After the GHHI program in-home modifications, did the children living at home miss school/daycare because of their asthma?

◯ Yes ◯ No

D-2. If yes, approximately how many days per month was asthma responsible for their missing school?

D-3. If yes, approximately how many days per month the child's/children's asthma caused adult(s) in the household to miss part of a day of work?

[ ]

D-3B. How many times per month did it cause adult(s) in the household to miss a full day of work?

[ ]

D-4. If yes, approximately how many times per month was asthma responsible for your taking the child/children to:

the clinic and/or urgent care

[ ]

the emergency room department

[ ]

asthma related hospitalizations

[ ]

D-5. How much money do you spend per month on asthma urgent care/ER visits/hospitalizations post GHHI program??

[ ]

D-6. Who bears health system cost for asthma ER visits/hospitalizations after the GHHI program?

○ Medicaid ○ Medicare ○ Private Insurance ○ Hospital ○ Self

D-7. After the GHHI program entered your home to make its changes, how are the child/children doing in school?

○ not well ○ well ○ good ○ very good

D-8. Do you believe that the GHHI program

○ helped you
○ didn't affect you positively or negatively
○ had a negative impact on you and those with whom you live.

Is there anything else you would be willing to share with me about your feelings concerning the GHHI program?

[ ]

REFERENCES

[1] Georgia Asthma Surveillance Report, 2013. URL: http://dph.georgia.gov/sites/dph.georgia.gov/files/related_files/site_page/2014%20Asthma%20Prevalence%20Report.pdf.

[2] Strategic Plan for Addressing Asthma in Georgia, 2013. URL: http://dph.georgia.gov/sites/dph.georgia.gov/files/related_files/site_page/DPH%20Asthma%20Strategic%20Plan%20for%20Asthma%202013_2018%20Final.pdf.

[3] Pettignano R, Bliss LR, Caley SB, McLaren S. Can access to a medical-legal partnership benefit patients with asthma who live in an urban community? J Health Care Poor Underserved. 2013;24(706): 706-17.

[4] Brooks W. Telephone interview GHHI program manager. Atlanta, GA: Georgia State, 2014 Sept 2.

[5] 2011 Housing Profile: Atlanta-Sandy Springs-Marietta, GA. www.census.gov/ prod/2013pubs/ahs11-3.pdf.

[6] US Mayor Newspaper: Baltimore Green, Healthy Homes Initiative transforms low-Income communities. URL: http://usmayors.org/usmayornewspaper/documents/07_19_10/pg20_baltimore_bp.asp.

[7] Evaluation of the ZAP Asthma Project. URL: http://zapasthma.org/index.html. Accessed September 5, 2014.

[8] Rivlin AM, George M. Can we reduce childhood asthma and lower costs, too? URL: http://www.brookings.edu/blogs/up-front/posts/2014/11/12-asthma-payment-reform-policyrivlin?utm_campaign=Brookings+Brief&utm_source=hs_email&utm_medium=email&utm_content=14881937&_hsenc=p2ANqtznBJKTMNq6hUVGC51dYZ47-LY_UtIv0w4AcgAodgShPDRvkocmRJT5Z7o4fRtLhK1YMpm566kZeB_8jA0nc O2X4W6Q&_hsmi=14881937.

[9] Bhaumik U, Norris K, Charron G, Walker SP, Sommer SJ, Chan E, et al. A cost analysis for a community-based case management intervention program for pediatric asthma. J Asthma 2013;50(3):310–7.

In: Environmental Health Disparities
Editors: I Leslie Rubin and Joav Merrick

ISBN: 978-1-63484-211-2

Chapter 10

THE FAMILY CHECK-UP IN A PEDIATRIC CLINIC AND BEHAVIOR IN THE HOME ENVIRONMENT

S Courtney Smith**, *Karen E Schetzina, Jodi Polaha, Katie Baker and David Wood
Department of Psychology, East Tennessee State University, Johnson City, Tennessee,
Department of Pediatrics, Quillen College of Medicine,
East Tennessee State University, Johnson City,
Tennessee and College of Public Health,
East Tennessee State University, Johnson City, Tennessee, US

In this chapter, we examine the feasibility of adapting the Family Check Up (FCU), an evidence-based program to identify and manage behavioral concerns in children ages 4 and 5 years, within a pediatric primary care clinic with an integrated mental health professional. Methods: Caregivers attending their child's 4 and 5 year-old well child visit were asked to complete a screening tool (Pediatric Symptom Checklist-17; PSC-17) measuring behavioral concerns as part of routine care. Families who screened positively, were referred to the FCU and asked to participate in a study evaluating the intervention. The FCU is a 2 session intervention during which information on home environment and parenting style was collected through tailored questionnaires, videotaped interactions, and a clinical interview. Feasibility was examined using portions of the Reach, Effectiveness, Adoption, Implementation, and Maintenance (REAIM) framework from the Dissemination and Implementation Science field. This study presents preliminary data on the domains of Reach and Adoption over the first 5 months of the FCU. Results: The number of families referred who attended at least one session (Reach) was 77.2%. Current data shows that use of the PSC-17 screening instrument (Adoption) is 91.4% for well child checks and 25% for acute visits. Adoption of those referred to the FCU is 84%, indicating most families screening positively for behavioral concerns were successfully referred to the FCU. Conclusion: Initial results suggest Reach and Adoption rates support the feasibility of adapting a behavioral intervention for delivery in the pediatric clinic. Notably, having an existing integrated care delivery model is a critical piece to this early

* Corresponding author: Ms. Courtney Smith, MA, Clinical Psychology Graduate Student, Department of Psychology, East Tennessee State University, POBox 70649, Tennessee, United States. E-mail: scourtneysmith@gmail.com.

success. Future directions will continue to explore feasibility of the remaining REAIM domains.

INTRODUCTION

The southern Appalachian region of the United States experiences a higher rate of health disparities compared to other parts of the nation; children are particularly vulnerable to adverse health outcomes. Specifically, children in this region have increased risks for lower birth weights (1), higher blood lead levels (2), higher rates of asthma (3) and poorer dental health (4). Behaviorally, children from the southern Appalachian region are more likely to lead sedentary lifestyles (5), have higher caloric diets (6), rates of obesity (7, 8) and more frequently engage in alcohol and substance abuse (9).

Parents from this area also report that their children have more behavioral and psychosocial problems compared to other regions of the United States. Parent reported behavioral concerns occur at a rate of 21% versus the national average of 10-14% (10). The higher rate of behavioral concerns in childhood is particularly concerning because problematic behaviors in children such as oppositional behavior (i.e., noncompliance) and conduct problems (i.e., physical aggression) are disturbingly predictive of negative outcomes in adolescence and early adulthood (11, 12). The following studies support the trajectory of continued behavioral and psychosocial issues that begin early in childhood and continue through adolescence into adulthood. One study reported that more than half of children who score positively on a measure of behavioral concerns at age 2 remain positive at age 5 years (11). Another study reported problematic behaviors exhibited at age 5 years are salient predictors of persistent conduct problems, such as aggression, through childhood (11, 12). Finally, Shaw, Gilliom and Giovanelli (13) found antisocial behaviors present in school-aged children are present through adolescence. If left untreated, children with behavioral problems are less likely to gain employment, or to remain employed, have less successful interpersonal and romantic partnerships, and have less effective parenting styles (14).

Furthermore, poor parenting styles can contribute to the development of behavioral concerns in children, negatively impacting their success as adults. The family and home environment in which a young child develops, contributes to his/her functioning as an adult. If their environment is unsupported in a way that inhibits healthy emotional and physical development children will fall into the cycle of disadvantage and disability with fewer opportunities to overcome their behavioral and psychosocial challenges. Figure 1 illustrates the point at which an insufficient home environment affects a child's trajectory and future generations.

Fortunately, there are many validated and effective behavioral interventions designed to target problematic behaviors, such as defiance and aggression, with the goal of improving a child's trajectory. Interventions with the most valid and reliable effects are those that are family-centered and target parenting styles (15), such as Parent-Child Interaction Therapy (16), The Incredible Years (17) and the Family Check-Up (18). Consistently praising positive behavior, ignoring mildly undesirable behavior, and providing transitions between activities encourage stronger bonds between parents and their children (19). These interventions emphasize the important role that proactive parenting plays in predicting improvement in conduct problems (20).

Unfortunately, few families become aware of these efficacious interventions, which are typically offered in traditional mental health settings. There are likely several reasons for this, each of which is heightened in rural Appalachia. First, there is stigma and negative attitudes associated with mental health services (21, 22). Second, mental health treatments are often too expensive and time-intensive for consistent participation and parents find it to be a cumbersome task (22). Finally, there is a significant shortage of mental health providers to deliver these services (22).

One method of overcoming the inaccessibility of evidence-based treatment is to offer services in alternate settings that are more familiar and comfortable for families. Indeed, family-centered interventions are evolving to move from engaging parents in traditional mental health clinical settings to community and school-based settings (23, 24). Interestingly, families are more likely to seek help for these concerns from their child's pediatrician rather than specialty mental health care services (10); therefore, it would be logical to develop a mechanism for delivering those interventions within a pediatric primary care clinic.

Placing an intervention in a primary care setting could eliminate issues for families, like locating a new mental or behavioral health site and traveling to that location. Further, the pediatrician would be closely involved with the referral process and the doctor-patient trust would be more easily transferred to a mental health professional working alongside the pediatrician.

The FCU is a validated intervention, endorsed by the National Institute of Drug Abuse, for children ages 2 through 17 to reduce rates of drug abuse, antisocial behavior, and depression (18, 25, 26). The FCU, designed to fit into three sessions, aims to achieve this goal by improving family management practices, particularly in families with high-risk environments (e.g., low socioeconomic status, history of family drug use). Additionally, the FCU targets parental variables that may also contribute to persistent problematic behavior, such as parental well-being, day-to-day parenting challenges, and low social support (27). Current parents with variables contributing to persistent behavior problems in their children likely lived in unhealthy home environments as children, illustrating the impact the health disparities cycle has from generation to generation in Figure 1. Compared to other family-centered interventions, the FCU differs by considering a health maintenance model, with a comprehensive assessment of family functioning, and by motivating change within parents (28, 20).

To evaluate the implementation of the FCU in a pediatric clinic the Reach, Effectiveness, Adoption, Implementation and Maintenance (REAIM) model will be used (30, 31). REAIM offers a framework for systematically evaluating various facets of an intervention in a clinical setting. This paper will only focus on the domains of Reach and Adoption (see Table 1). Reach refers to the percentage of patients referred to the FCU and Adoption examines the percentage of those screening positive on questionnaire that were referred to the FCU.

The aim of this study was to evaluate the initial implementation and feasibility of the FCU via an integrated delivery care procedure, in a primary care pediatric clinic that serves a health disparate population located in northeastern Tennessee. It is hypothesized that preliminary results will indicate high rates of Reach and Adoption.

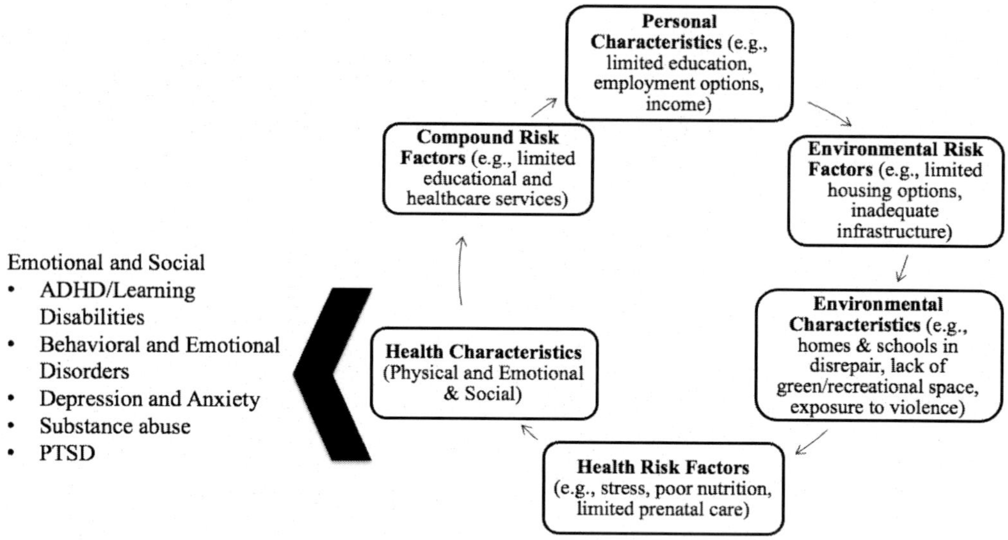

Figure 1. Adapted from "Break the Cycle 10" diagram of health disparities 2015.

Table 1. REAIM domain definitions (italicized domains were the focus of this paper)

Domains	Definition
Reach	*What percentage of referred families are willing to attend the FCU?*
Effectiveness	Do parents report improved child behavior/decrease risk following the FCU?
Adoption	*What percentage of "at-risk" 4 and 5 year-olds are referred to the FCU by their pediatrician?*
Implementation	Can the FCU be implemented with fidelity?
Maintenance	Is the FCU financially sustainable in this setting?

OUR STUDY

The FCU was implemented at a primary care pediatric clinic located in northeastern Tennessee in early 2015. One psychologist and three doctoral level psychology students worked as behavioral health consultants (BHC) providing integrated care at the pediatric clinic and who were trained in the delivery of the FCU at the University of Oregon.

Although the FCU is a relatively short 3-session, evidence-based intervention compared to lengthier programs that require a several week commitment (e.g., Parent-Child Interaction Therapy, Triple P), it still remains a cumbersome process to fit into a primary care setting; therefore, the FCU was adapted to fit the clinic flow and infrastructure. To begin, the FCU was made to fit into two sessions, instead of the requisite three (see Figure 2). This was made possible by working closely with the developers to identify the critical components of the intervention and excluding non-essential components. The final adapted intervention included an assessment process with multiple sources of input (i.e., questionnaires, video-taped interactions, clinical interview), use of an ecological approach to family functioning, identification of a collaborative set between parents and therapist, motivational interviewing, and use of a pre-existing form designed to frame feedback. It is characteristically individualized, flexible, utilizes SMART-goals, and can be conducted across two, possibly three sessions (see Table 2). Next, an optimal space within the clinic was identified to conduct the FCU thus avoiding examination room congestion. Finally, video technology via GoPro and a computer tablet was utilized to capture footage of parent-child interactions to be utilized in the final session.

To achieve a high level of adoption, the practice personnel (i.e., administrators, nurses, and pediatricians) were closely involved in assisting in the development of an efficient protocol, which would not disrupt clinic flow and efficiency. Once all the delivery components were decided upon, all providers and staff were informed of the implementation plan within the clinic and trained on their respective roles. The roles of the administrative staff, nurses, and pediatricians entailed: 1) ensuring all families with children attending their 4 and 5 year-old well child visit received a Pediatric Symptom Checklist -17 (PSC-17) - this measure fits on a one page document and was printed on green paper for ease of recognition; 2) scoring the PSC-17, to be calculated by pediatrician; 3) referring families to the FCU (if they screened positively on the PSC-17 then they were introduced to the FCU, and encouraged to follow through with a referral to the on-site Behavioral Health Consultant (BHC), i.e., a clinical psychology doctoral student), and; 4) helping with scheduling future FCU appointments.

If a family screened positively in the PSC-17, the pediatrician presented the FCU behavioral service offered in the clinic and referred them to the BHC for the FCU and they either: 1) met with a BHC during that visit via a 'warm hand-off' (a process by which the primary care provider directly introduces the family to the BHC at the time of the child's medical visit), and began the first session of the FCU; 2) met with the BHC via a warm hand-off and scheduled the first FCU session for a later date due to scheduling considerations; 3) or scheduled a separate appointment without meeting the BHC to begin the first session. Finally, caregivers were asked if they were willing to have information collected (e.g., data from the PSC-17, videotaped interactions) from the FCU be included in a research study evaluating this intervention (see Figures 2 and 3). This study had Institutional Review Board approval.

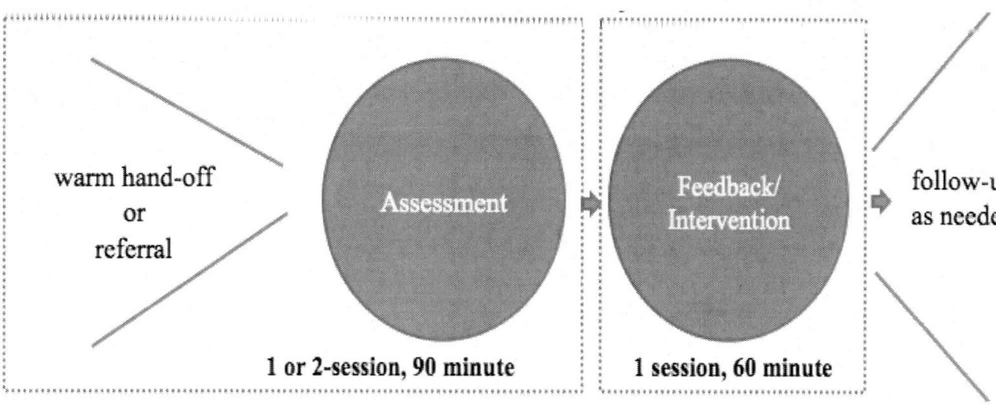

Figure 2. Adapted family check-up for the pediatric primary care clinic.

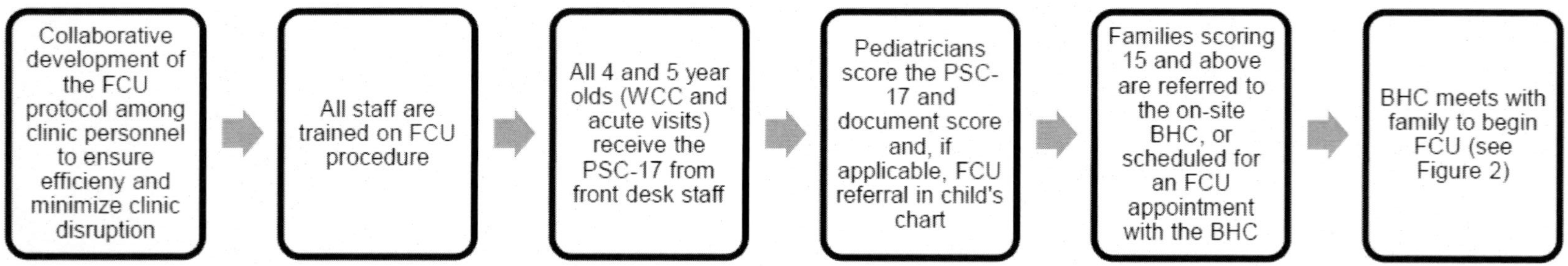

Figure 3. FCU development and implementation process.

Table 2. Core components of the adapted family check-up

Assessment has multiple input sources - interview questionnaires, videotaped interactions, clinical interview
Ecological Approach (across all components)
Collaborative Set and Strength Focused (to occur during the Interview and Feedback sessions)
Motivational Interviewing (Feedback session)
Use of Feedback Form to frame discussion
Flexible, Individualized, SMART-style goal setting

The PSC-17 is a 17-item measure for caregivers of children, which consists of internalizing, externalizing and inattention subscales. Caregivers rate each item as either "often," "sometimes," or "never" present in a child. Each response is assigned a value of 2, 1, or 0, respectively. The responses are added together to yield both a subscale score and a total score. A positive score is considered when the PSC-17 total score is 15 or greater (32).

A record list for all 4 and 5 year-old well-child checks (WCC) from January 2015 through June 2015 was obtained. In February, due to initial low enrollment, the study was expanded to also include all 4 and 5 year-old acute visits. Therefore, acute records lists were from February 2015 to June 2015. Each child's records were located in the electronic health record (EHR).

Each child's record was checked for the following information in order to assess Reach and Adoption of the FCU. 1) Was the visit a WCC or an acute visit? 2) Was the PSC-17 given to the family? 3) What was the PSC-17 score? 4) Did the child score ≥ 15? 5) Was the child referred to the FCU? 6) How many sessions of the FCU were attended by the family if the child was referred to the FCU? These data were obtained by the Office of Information Technology, then stored, managed, and analyzed by a research assistant. The protocol and informed consent was approved by East Tennessee State University's Institutional Review Board.

Table 3. Results of reach and adoption

Domain	N	Percentage
Reach	**22**	
Session 1	17	77.2%
Session 2	6	27.2%
Session 3	3	13.6%
Adoption	**281**	
PSC-17		
WCC (N = 164)	150	91%
Acute Visits (N = 117)	29	25%
FCU ≥ 15	**19**	
FCU Referrals	16	84%

FINDINGS

The clinic generally serves families from low-income households holding state Medicaid insurance plans (approximately 85%); however, this specific information was not collected for the purposes of this project. A review of the electronic health records showed 281 4- and 5-year-old WCC (n = 164) and acute (n = 117) appointments occurred between the months of January and June. Ninety-one percent (n = 150) of families attending WCC and 25% (n = 29) of those attending an acute visit were given and completed the PSC-17, as noted in each chart. Seven percent (n = 19) of all families scored their child ≥15. In terms of adopting the FCU, 84% (n = 16) of families who score ≥ 15 were referred, by their pediatrician, to the FCU. In addition to families who met criteria for the study, there were six additional FCU referrals (i.e., families who scored <15) made to the FCU by the pediatricians based on clinical judgment (see table 3). To date, 77.2% (17 of 22) of families referred attended at least one session, 27.2% (n = 6) attended at least two sessions, and 13.6% (n = 3) attended 3 sessions.

DISCUSSION

This study examined the preliminary implementation of the FCU within a pediatric primary care clinic to address behavioral concerns that commonly arise in pediatric visits. This study utilized the REAIM model to evaluate the real-world application of the FCU. REAIM outlines domains that are important to consider when evaluating the sustainability of an intervention.

At this time, only two of the five domains were used in the current evaluation (i.e., Reach and Adoption). Reach measured the number of participants who were willing to participate in the intervention. Results indicated a little over three quarters of families who score positive on the PSC-17 chose to begin treatment by attending at least one session. The first session included brief education about the FCU and signing an informed consent. After the first session, however, Reach decreased and only one-quarter of families followed-up with the second visit with even fewer attending the final session, if there was one scheduled. The time between each session was approximately one week. However, some of this decrease is due to future appointments that have yet to happen and not included in this rate. There was no follow-up with families who did not attend scheduled appointments.

The rates of Reach for the first visit exceeded the rate of FCU Reach in school settings by nearly 50%; however, the decrease in subsequent visits is consistent with previous reports (33). The decrease in participation could be due to a variety of reasons. For example, even 2 additional visits may be too difficult for families, or perhaps a brief discussion with a mental health professional concluded in some non-specific therapeutic effects that improved parental perception of their child's behaviors. Conversely, after the first session some families may have felt the service would not be helpful for their concerns. Information regarding why families failed to attend follow-up visits could provide information useful to improving the delivery of the program.

Adoption measured two components of the FCU. First, it measured the percentage of patients who received the PSC-17. Results indicated there was a high Adoption rate of the PSC-17 at the WCC and a much lower rate of Adoption for the acute visits, even when controlling for acute visits start date. Since the inclusion of 4 and 5 year acute visits was made about a month post-implementation, the front desk might not have remembered to hand out the PSC-17 to every 4 and 5 year-old visit (WCC or acute). This discrepancy could also be due to the fact that pediatricians were not initially trained or expected to screen for behavioral concerns using the PSC-17 during acute visits; therefore, assessing for behavioral concerns was not a priority if, for example, a child only presented with an ear infection. Anecdotal evidence suggests some pediatricians suggest acute visits do not typically include routine screening and instead have a targeted concern; therefore, it can be challenging to remember to incorporate the behavioral measure, especially for a specific age range and not every child. Although, if the staff training initially considered including acute visits there may have been opportunity to brainstorm with medical staff on how to best incorporate the PSC-17 as routine practice for acute visits.

Second, Adoption also measured the percentage of FCU referrals. Pediatricians successfully referred a high percentage of all families with positive scores for their child's behavior on the PSC-17. However, there is room for improvement, since the intended goal was to have *every* positively screening child referred to the FCU.

Overall, the initial Reach and Adoption of the FCU appears promising and supports the feasibility of implementing an evidence-based treatment in an established primary care clinic across at least these two domains. It is also important to note the components that likely contributed to the FCU's initial success. First and foremost, this particular clinic supports, and operates as, an integrated model of care that includes the presence of an onsite mental health professional. In this case the mental health professionals were masters-level clinical psychology doctoral students who were closely supervised by a licensed clinical psychologist. The initial data support that many children are being screened and receiving intervention for behavioral problems who might otherwise escape treatment.

There are three apparent limitations of this evaluation of the FCU and the results. First, generalizability should be pursued with caution. The FCU was only implemented and evaluated within one pediatric clinic. Further, the clinic in which it was implemented was primed and groomed to anticipate procedural changes in patient care as best practices evolve due to its nature as a medical and health professional training location, and there may have already been a level of operational and procedural flexibility that might not otherwise exist in other clinics.

Second, the FCU is an intervention that is intended to work for children of all ages. For this study the FCU was only applied to children ages 4 and 5. It may be the case that using this intervention on children of different ages may yield a different FCU follow-through rate or be more effective evoking changes in the child's behavior. Finally, future studies will examine the remaining domains of the REAIM framework, which will provide a deeper understanding of the feasibility of the intervention in a primary care clinic.

REFERENCES

[1] Hulme PA, Belgen MA. Residential status and birth outcomes: Is rural/urban distinction adequate? Public Health Nurs 1999;16:176–81.

[2] Schaffer SJ, Kincaid MS, Endres J. Lead poisoning risk determination in a rural setting. Pediatr 1996;97:84-90.

[3] Ernst P, Cormier Y. Relative scarcity of asthma and atopy among rural adolescents raised on a farm. Am J Respir Crit Care Med 2000;16:1563-66.
[4] Vargas CM, Monajemy N, Khurana P, Tinanoff N. Oral health status of children attending Head Start Maryland. Pediatr Dent 2000;24:257-63.
[5] Hortz B, Stevens E, Holden B, Petosa RL. Rates of physical activity among rural Appalachian adolescents in Ohio. J Rural Health 2000;25:58-61.
[6] Crooks DL. Food consumption, activity, and overweight among elementary school children in an Appalachian Kentucky Community. Am J Phys Anthropol 2000; 112:159-70.
[7] Centers for Disease Control and Prevention. Estimated county-level prevalence of diabetes and obesity United States, 2007. MMWR 2009;58:1259-63.
[8] Lutifyya MN, Lipsky MS, Wisdom-Behounek J, Inpanbutr-Martinkus M. Is rural residency a risk factor for overweight and obesity in U.S. children? Obes 2007;15:2348-56.
[9] Johnson AO, Mink MD, Harun N, Moore CG, Martin AB, Bennett KJ. Violence and drug use in rural teens: National prevalence estimates from the 2003 youth risk behavior survey. J Sch Health 2008;78:554-61.
[10] Polaha J, Dalton W, Allen S. The prevalence of emotional and behavior problems in pediatric primary care serving rural children. J Pediatr Psychol 2011;36:652-60.
[11] Campbell SB, Shaw DS, Gilliom, M. Early externalizing behavior problems: Toddlers and preschoolers at risk for later maladjustment. Dev Psychopathol 2000;12:467-88.
[12] Shaw DS, Bell RQ, Gilliom M. A truly early starter model of antisocial behavior revisited. Clin Child Fam Psychol Rev 2000;3:155-72.
[13] Shaw DS, Gilliom M, Giovannelli J. Aggressive behavior disorders. In: Zeanah CH, eds. Handbook of infant mental health, 2nd ed. New York: Guilford, 2000:397-411.
[14] Coie, J, Dodge, K. Aggression and antisocial behavior. In: Damon W, Eisenberg N, eds. Handbook of child psychology fifth edition. Hoboken, NJ: John Wiley, 1998;3:779-862.
[15] Conduct Problem Prevention Research Group. Evaluation of the first 3 years of the Fast Track Prevention Trial with children at high risk for adolescent conduct problem. J Abnorm Child Psychol 2002;30:19-35.
[16] Nixon CB, Sweeney L, Erikson, DB, Touyz SW. Parent-child interaction therapy: A comparison of standard and abbreviated treatments for oppositional defiant preschoolers. J Consult Clin Psychol 2003;71:251-60.
[17] Webster-Stratton C. Advancing videotape parent training: A comparison study. J Consult Clin Psychol 1998;66:715-30.
[18] Dishion TJ, Nelson NE, Kavanagh K. The Family Check-Up with high-risk young adolescents: Preventing early onset substance use by parent monitoring. Behav Ther 2003;34;553-71.
[19] Sugai G, Horner RH, Sprague JR. Functional-assessment-based behavior support planning: Research to practice to research. Behav Disord 1999;24: 223-7.
[20] Gardner F, Ward S, Burton J, Wilson C. Joint play and the early development of conduct problems in children: A longitudinal observational study of preschoolers. Soc Dev 2003;12:361-79.
[21] Goldsmith HF, Wagenfeld MO, Manderscheid RW, Stiles D. Specialty mental health services in metropolitan and nonmetropolitan areas: 1983 and 1990. Adm Policy Ment Health 1997;24:475–88.
[22] U.S. Department of Health and Human Services, Health Resources and Services Administration. (2005). Mental health and rural America: 1994–2005. Rockville, MD: Office of Rural Health Policy. Boyd MR & Mackey MC (2000). Running away to nowhere: Rural women's experiences of becoming alcohol dependent. Arch Psychiatr Nurs 2000;14(3):142-149.
[23] Baker CN, Arnold, DH, Meagher S. Enrollment and attendance in a parent training prevention program for conduct problems. Prev Sci 2011;12:126-38.
[24] Gardner F, Burton J, Klimes I. Randomized controlled trial of a parenting intervention in the voluntary sector for reducing child conduct problems. J Child Psychol Psychiatry 2006;47:1123-32.
[25] Dishion TJ, ed. Universal family-centered prevention strategies: Current findings and critical issues for public health impact. Prev Sci, 2002;3;191-201.
[26] Connell A, Dishion, TJ. Reducing depression among at-risk early adolescent: Three-year effects of a family-centered intervention embedded within schools. J Fam Psychol 2008:22:574-85.

[27] Dishion TJ, Stormshak EA, Kavanagh K. Everyday parenting: A professional's guide to building family management skills. Champaign, IL: Research Press, 2012.

[28] Bullock BM, Forgatch MS. Mothers in transition: Model-based strategies for effective parenting. In: Pinso WM, Lebow JL, eds. Family psychology: The art of the science. New York: Oxford University Press, 2005;349-71.

[29] Gill AM, Luke WH, Shaw DS, Dishion TJ, Wilson MN. The family check-up in early childhood: A case study of intervention process and change. J Clin Child Adolesc Psychol 2008;37:893-904.

[30] Brownson RC, Colditz GA, Procotor EK. Dissemination and implementation research in health: Translating science to practice. New York: Oxford University Press, 2012.

[31] Glasgow R, Vogt T, Boles S. Evaluating the public health impact of health promotion interventions: the REAIM framework. Am J Public Health 1999;89:1322-7.

[32] Gardner W, Campo J, Lucas A. Validation of the PSC-17 in a primary care sample. Pediatr Res 2004;55:242A-43A.

[33] Connell A, Dishion, TJ, Yasui, M, Kavanagh, K. An adaptive approach to family intervention: Linking engagement in family centered intervention to reductions in adolescent problem behavior. J Consult Clin Psychol 2007;75:568-79.

In: Environmental Health Disparities
Editors: I Leslie Rubin and Joav Merrick

ISBN: 978-1-63484-211-2

Chapter 11

EXERCISE AND HEALTHY EATING: MULTI-LEVEL COMMUNITY BASED INTERVENTION

Naeemah Ruffin*[*], *Sharon Levine and Cappy Collins
Icahn School of Medicine at Mount Sinai, New York,
New York, US

A community-based intervention (Concrete Safaris) in East Harlem that operates on three levels (the individual, the neighborhood, and public policy) to enable children to exercise and eat a healthy diet will improve their fitness levels and can lead to improved academic performance. Methods: Cohort study in two phases: Phase 1 assesses academic performance, school attendance and improvement in fitness of all students enrolled in the Concrete Safaris program from both school years 2012-2013 and 2013-2014. This phase is focused on assessing the utilization of the program by the participants in the first and second year of the Concrete Safaris program. Phase 2 assesses academic performance, school attendance and improvement in fitness of the students in the Concrete Safaris program comparing them to a control group of students selected from the school district who are not enrolled in the Concrete Safaris program. Results: Preliminary Phase 1 results demonstrate that consistent enrollment in the Concrete Safaris program by students returning from the previous year both improved their fitness and raised their academic performance. Discussion: A child's environment, both in the home and outside the home, can positively or negatively affect the child's ability to improve his or her conscious decision-making skills and default healthy behaviors that will positively impact his or her life. Changing a child's environment through a multi-level, community-based intervention, can enable the child to be healthy and live life to the fullest. This study is based on assessing the effectiveness of this type of intervention.

[*] Corresponding author: Naeemah Ruffin, DPM/MPH Candidate, Icahn School of Medicine at Mount Sinai and New York College of Podiatric Medicine, New York, United States. E-mail: naeemahruffin@yahoo.com.

INTRODUCTION

The United States Census Bureau predicts that racial and ethnic minority populations in the U.S. will grow to become half of the U.S. population in three decades (1). A review of health statistics of low-income communities across America such as the East Harlem community in Manhattan, New York City, demonstrates that the children in this population live in an environment that makes it difficult for them to thrive. From an economic perspective having a healthy population contributing to society is a key factor to the future prosperity of America. A key step in ensuring a healthy population is to provide children with the tools they need to improve their conscious decision-making skills and default healthy behaviors which tend to be based on social norms.

There is increasing research that shows the risk for childhood and adolescent obesity appears during the early childhood years (2). Children who tend to have a high BMI, are overweight, or obese in early childhood, are more likely to be overweight or obese in later in childhood and in their teens (2). Therefore, eating and physical activity habits developed early in childhood are likely important and may determine the weight trajectory over a child's lifetime.

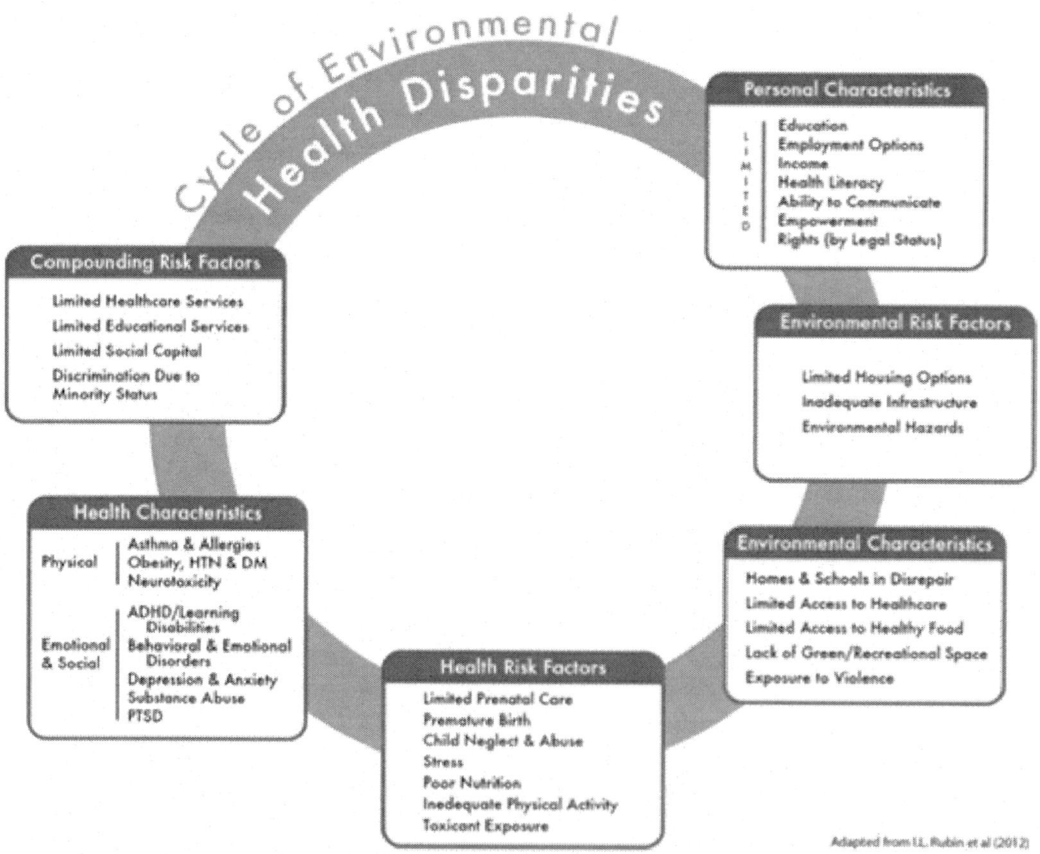

Figure 1. Cycle of environmental health disparities.

Children age 17 years and under make up about 28% of the population in East Harlem which represents a higher proportion than in Manhattan (17%), and overall in New York City (NYC) (24%) (3). Compared with children nationwide, almost 40% of NYC children are overweight (18% in NYC vs. 14% nationwide) and obese (21% in NYC vs. 17% nationwide)(4). Exploring these obesity statistics more deeply by gender and race, from kindergarten to 8th grade in NYC, boys are more likely to be obese than girls (24% vs. 19%). This difference is seen across racial and ethnic groups, except among Black students for whom there is no difference between boys and girls (21% obese). With regard to race, it was noted that Hispanic students are the most affected with 29% of Hispanic boys being obese (4).

These health disparities among the East Harlem children are driven by a variety of interrelated risk factors that have been described by Rubin et al. (5) as a "cycle of environmental health disparities" (see Figure 1). These risk factors can be categorized as those that affect the individual, the community, and public policy. For example, the factors affecting the individual can occur inside the home such as parental values and cultural influences impacting food choices; environmental factors outside the home at a community level can affect the accessibility to healthy food and the availability of green spaces for physical activity; and structural barriers are factors occurring at the public policy level.

At the individual level, parental values and cultural influences have a tremendous impact on the health of a child. The choices a child makes later in life are influenced largely by their home and community environment. Remarkably, 31% of the adults in East Harlem are obese and 31% are overweight which is the highest proportion of obese adults among all neighborhoods in New York City (3). Furthermore, the parents' cultural values and attitudes also may play a role in a child's weight. For example, a study conducted among Latino families in Brooklyn, NY suggests that parents and grandparents are often very pleased with the appearance of an overweight or obese child or grandchild, particularly toddlers (6). Some Latino mothers believe that more weight on a child makes the child more physically protected than a child who is slim (6). Also, many Latino mothers do not believe that the additional weight of their children who are overweight or obese will have a significant impact on their health long-term and weight problems can be overcome when the child becomes an adult (6).

Children in East and Central Harlem have minimal access to healthy foods. The lack of healthy food choices is driven by the type of food available in the East Harlem neighborhood. For example, fast-food establishments are more prevalent than restaurants with healthy foods in East and Central Harlem than in the upper middle class neighborhood of the Upper East Side (7). Complicating this situation is when low-income families do not have enough money to purchase healthy food for the family, they may take on unhealthy eating habits in hopes of stretching the food budget (2). This may lead them to buy low-cost, energy-dense, nutrient-deficient foods that will have a higher content of fat and sugar and a lower content of vital nutrients (2). Access to affordable, nutritious foods that are not heavily processed, such as fresh fruits and vegetables, and foods rich in vitamins and fiber may make it easier for children to maintain a healthy weight. Additionally, poor nutrition can impact academic performance by affecting the capacity to learn, grow, and develop. This influence can start as early as conception and continue throughout childhood and into adulthood (8, 9). Research continues to support the fact that proper nutrition early in life can affect cognitive performance later in life. This becomes an important consideration especially when designing public health food policy.

Physical activity in children is crucial for neurodevelopment (10-12). Therefore, lack of access to green spaces for children to play and promote physical activity can be detrimental to a child's health and achievement. What is key to understanding the causes of the lack of green spaces is appreciating how the community is designed. East Harlem is a built environment comprised of brownstones and small apartment buildings, commercial areas, high-rise housing complexes, large institutions and super block developments (13,14). East Harlem has the highest concentration of public housing developments in New York City (13). Thirty percent of the East Harlem population lives in public housing and the New York City Housing Authority (NYCHA) property totals 13.5% of the total land area (13). These developments consist of tall, bulky buildings surrounded by open green areas, often on super blocks which are developments that span several blocks requiring the closing of through streets. Excluding Randall's Island (see Figure 2), there is 0.7 acres of parkland per 1000 residents. 90% to 100% of the open space in the parkland contains impervious ground cover, such as pavement or rubber safety surfaces (13).

In one study, "Growing up healthy in East Harlem," 324 children were assessed in terms of how much time they spent outdoors per week and how much time they spent sedentary per day. The results revealed that they spent only 2 hours per week outdoors and 3 hours per day sedentary (15). Furthermore, more than half of teens in specific disadvantaged neighborhoods of East and Central Harlem (54%–64%) report an excess amount of time (three or more hours per school day) viewing television (16). Daily attendance at a physical education (PE) class is less common among teens in these neighborhoods than other NYC neighborhoods and teens in East and Central Harlem are nearly three times less likely to attend a daily PE class (16%) than other NYC teens who do not live in the East and Central Harlem neighborhoods (45%) (16).

Environmental and policy structural barriers make it even more challenging to impact factors inside and outside the home. These structural systems include institutions that involve the distribution of wealth, power, and resources over which an individual has no control (8). Ultimately, these systems can affect the living environment of individuals including their economic and social environment and access to health and social services (9). This situation in which an individual has no control over the circumstances in which one is born into and is shaped by broader economic, social, and political forces has been called the social determinants of health by the World Health Organization (17). Examples of structural barriers in East Harlem is the more than 100 acres of New York City Housing Authority (NYCHA) open space that is fenced off and inaccessible to residents (18). In addition, East Harlem residents do not have adequate access to nearby Randall's Island, a major nearby park for the community. These structural barriers have broad reaching effects on the health of the children in these communities.

Since the above factors exist at multiple levels and are interrelated, it becomes challenging to address any one or more of these factors with a singularly-focused intervention. Is there an intervention that could work on multiple levels (the individual, the neighborhood, and public policy) to enable children to exercise regularly and eat a healthy diet, thereby improving their academic performance and overall fitness?

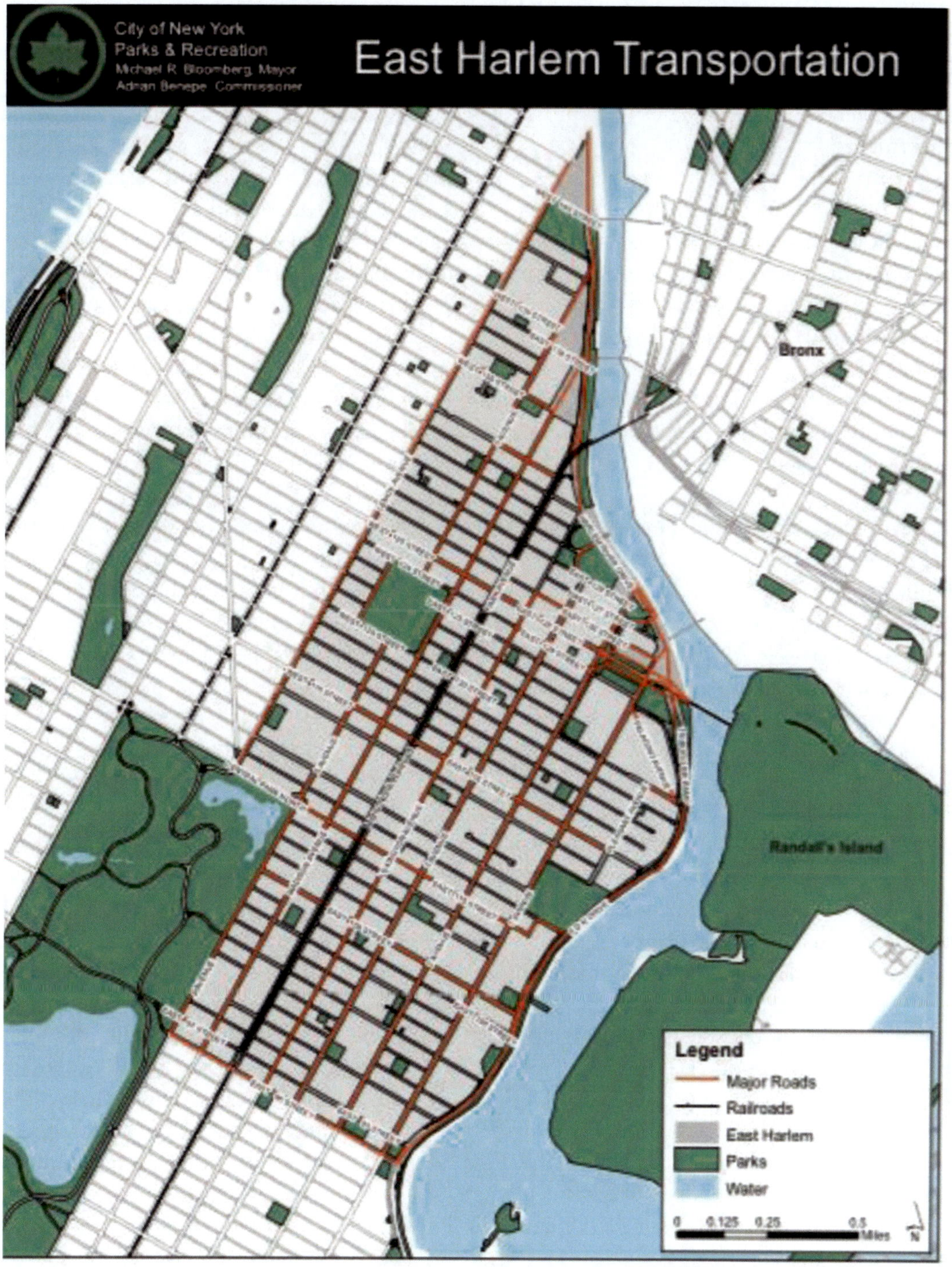

Figure 2. Note: Randall's Island is excluded from the East Harlem Community.

LITERATURE REVIEW

A literature review was performed to determine the best practices to enable children to exercise and eat a healthy diet to improve their fitness levels leading to improved academic performance.

There were ten community-based garden interventions (2, 19-26) that were reviewed. Two of these studies were quantitative (2, 19) and eight were qualitative (20-26). Both quantitative interventions consisted of community garden-based interventions. One intervention targeted 95 low-income Latino immigrant families and included a weekly gardening session, a 7-week cooking and nutrition workshop, and social events for parents and children (2). The results showed that 17% of obese or overweight children had improved their BMI classification and 100% of the children with a BMI classification of normal had maintained that BMI classification. The parents reported an increase of 146% in the availability of fruits and vegetables with a 28% increase in the consumption of fruits and 33% increase in the consumption of vegetables among children of families participating in this program (2).

However, the other quantitative intervention which consisted of an after-school gardening and nutrition curriculum covering eight lessons (n = 12 experimental, n = 21 control) revealed no differences in nutrition knowledge scores between or within groups at baseline or at the end of the program (19). It is believed that this was primarily due to the fact that for the population that was selected, the baseline scores were high for both groups. Furthermore, it was unclear which aspects of gardening (i.e., season, harvesting, crops grown) had the greatest impact on influencing the outcomes (19).

Of the seven qualitative studies that were reviewed, four reported positive results in influencing healthy eating habits among children (20-23). These consisted of two interventions located within organizations such as a children's garden at the Brooklyn Botanical Gardens (n = 10) (20) and a food garden at the North Bay Children's Center (NBCC) (23), a not-for profit early childhood education program in Marin County, California (n = 15). One intervention consisted of a community-based intervention targeted at the youth in Minneapolis, MN (n = 66) (21) which consisted of nutrition and cooking, and gardening classes and the last intervention consisted of a school garden (22).

There were two studies that reported mixed results (21, 24). The first study performed a review of the psychosocial basis of food to determine the best approach to positively influence a child's food choices (24). This study concluded that a 'one size fits all' approach to intervention design may not work well in all settings (24). What would contribute to positive results for a school gardening intervention is to tailor the message with reinforcement messaging, peer modeling, changing the food in the cafeteria and vending machines in schools, and repeated hands-on experiences such as planting and harvesting (24).

The second study that reported mixed results was a community-based intervention in Texas that consisted of a one-week summer camp format taking place once per week for twelve weeks in which participants were exposed to nutrition education and gardening activities (21). The effectiveness of the intervention was assessed via a questionnaire. The results of the study showed that there were no improvements in fruit and vegetable preferences but there were improvements in healthful snack consumption and knowledge about the benefits of eating fruits and vegetables (21). While these results were reported, it was unclear from this study which of the intervention formats were most effective: the 1-week summer camp or the once per week for 12 weeks intervention. It was also unclear which activities were more effective.

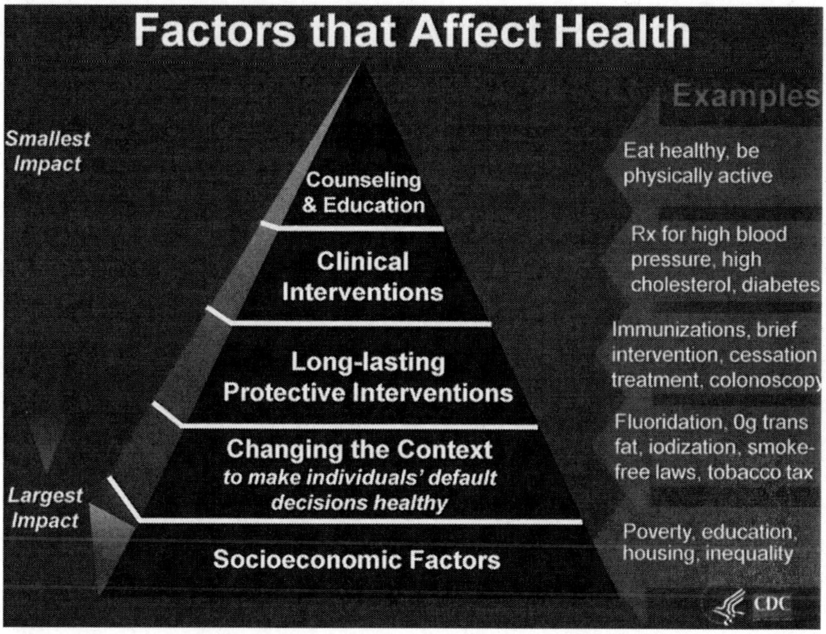

Figure 3. Frieden health impact pyramid.

While some of the literature describing community-based interventions suggests that school gardening programs can provide an interactive environment with the potential to change children's fruit and vegetable intake, the results reveal very little evidence to support the claims that school gardening alone can improve children's daily fruit and vegetable intake (25). Also, another study cited that interventions that target the homes of families may be more effective in improving fruit and vegetable access but may not demonstrate a significant impact (26).

Additional studies suggest strong evidence that link healthy eating habits and physical activity with academic achievement (27). For example, studies have suggested that the lack of adequate consumption of certain foods, such as fruits, vegetables, or dairy products is associated with lower grades among students. (28-30). Additionally, other studies suggest that students who are physically active tend to have better grades, school attendance, cognitive performance such as memory, and classroom behaviors (31-37).

On the other hand, some sources suggest a multi-level approach may be a more effective way to address health disparities resulting from socioeconomic determinants. For example, one study found that there are multiple factors, both upstream and downstream, that can impact fruit and vegetable consumption in a community. It is believed that the interventions that are upstream can reach past the individual level and impact the food availability and consumption at a population level (26). This view is also in line with the Frieden Health Impact Pyramid (see Figure 3) (38). The Frieden Health Impact Pyramid which is a 5-tier pyramid, illustrates the impact of different types of public health interventions that seek to provide a framework to best improve health (38). The base of the pyramid shows interventions with the greatest potential impact such as ones that address socioeconomic determinants of health. As you move up the pyramid the interventions become more individual-based such as education and counseling. This pyramid shows that interventions can exist on multiple levels and can have a varying impact. Also, implementing a single intervention that addresses multiple levels can achieve a maximum health impact (38).

Similarly, The National Institutes of Health (NIH) has reported that health promotion interventions require more than providing an education to individuals about ways to be healthy (39). Interventions should include strategies and programs that change individual's behavior along with making changes in the physical and social environment of the community at large (39). Strategies that target the community can include economic incentives that advocate for policies that support health (39).

Furthermore, a review of the best intervention strategies to increase the consumption of fruits and vegetables from the 2010 Center for Disease Control (CDC) guide suggests increasing access, availability, and consumption of fruits and vegetables (40). The proposed strategies can include "the use of food policy councils" to increase access to supermarkets and fresh fruit and vegetable markets, develop programs for schools and communities that grow food locally, improve access to fruits and vegetables at the workplace and in institutions of learning, support and promote neighborhood and home gardens by working with zoning and community development departments to convert vacant lots into gardens, develop policies to encourage healthy eating habits, such as fruit and vegetable consumption in schools through the availability of fruit and vegetables in the cafeteria and in vending machines (40). The creation of various advocacy channels will enable the community to express their needs and concerns to policymakers, economic and community development officials to improve the food environment (40).

Recommendation

Based on the literature review, it appears that to be effective in enabling children to exercise and eat a healthy diet to improve their fitness levels and improve academic performance, the intervention should address the multiple-levels of influence. Specifically, the intervention should connect the ecological aspect of the child's physical and social environment including changes in city and/or local government policies to more constructive policies enabling underserved communities to improve their conscious decision-making skills and default healthy behaviors. The ideal intervention should work on 3 levels: the individual, the community, and public policy.

For example, on a public policy level the intervention will need to work with local governmental agencies to create public policies that improve the ecological environment of low-income and underserved communities to reduce the overall societal risk factors contributing to disease and lower academic performance. Examples of these public policies would be to create a new infrastructure to improve neighborhoods and communities by creating green spaces and providing access to healthy food. On a neighborhood and community level, the public policy changes can lead to community-based partnership initiatives that help to improve neighborhoods through a focus on urban farming or gardens to provide better food to low-income neighborhoods that are typically deprived of supermarkets that sell healthy fruits and vegetables. And lastly, on an individual level community organizers can educate children and families on the importance of implementing a healthy lifestyle to reduce their individual risk factors for diseases.

Break the cycle

We have chosen to study the effectiveness of an intervention that works on multiple levels to break the cycle of environmental health disparities in a low-income neighborhood (see Figure 4). The intervention, Concrete Safaris, is a community-based organization with the mission of "providing youth with the experiential education to become environmental leaders and health advocates for themselves and their communities" (41). The outcomes of interest include health measures such as obesity, fitness and dietary habits, along with achievement measures such as academic performance (41). It achieves its mission by operating as an after-school program, designed in partnership with children living in East Harlem's public housing projects, to help improve academics, increase activity levels, increase calorie expenditure, and improve decision-making skills. Concrete Safaris is an intervention that is working on three levels: the individual, the neighborhood, and public policy. The key risk factors Concrete Safaris is focused on are highlighted in the "Cycle of Environmental Health Disparities" in (see Figure 4).

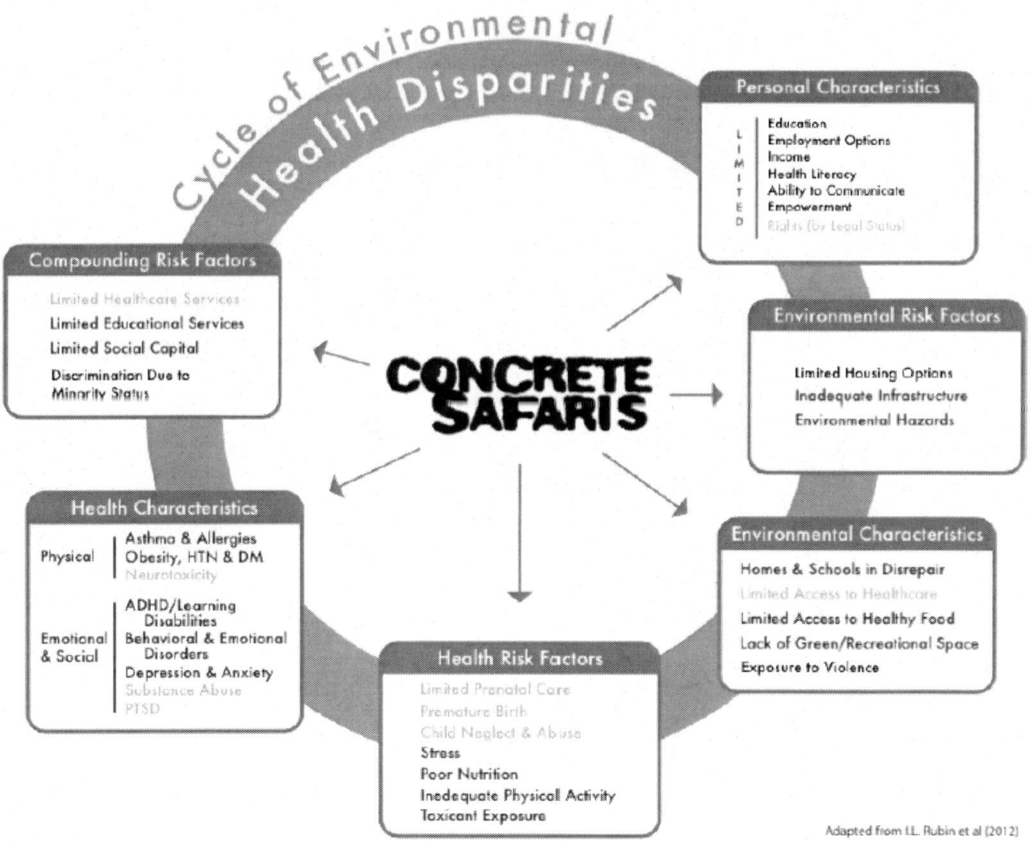

Figure 4.

Concrete Safaris partnered with Public School (P.S.) 102 in East Harlem to deliver a 5-day per week after school program in which children designed gardens, studied nutrition and cooked, developed bike routes and cycled those routes, and created an annual race to promote fitness among youth and families. Concrete Safaris along with its participants have met with the New York City Housing Authority (NYCHA) officials to secure land for gardens and then have grown thousands of pounds of produce, testified in favor of bike lanes in their neighborhood and then created bike routes, and outdoor activities for their community, and led workshops on health topics of their choosing (41). The program has been in operation for two full school years since 2012.

STUDY DESIGN

The study design is a cohort study to be performed in two phases. Phase one assesses academic performance, school attendance and improvement in fitness of all students enrolled and returning students in the Concrete Safaris program from the school years 2012-2013 and 2013-2014. Phase two assesses academic performance, school attendance and improvement in fitness of the students in the Concrete Safaris program comparing them to a matched control group of students selected from the same school district who are not enrolled in the Concrete Safaris program.

The setting of the program is in East Harlem (see Figure 2). The Concrete Safaris program design consists of a variety of weekly after school activities scheduled across each day of the school week (see Table 4). The activities for the 2013-2014 school year consisted of a nutrition workshop, gardening and landscaping, biking, science experiments/arts & crafts, and team building/concrete safaris challenge events. The activities for the 2012-2013 school year consisted of fitness, field trips, rugby, swimming, and gardening. Each activity lasts about 1.5 hours starting after school on each of the five days of the school week. The participants meet at P.S. 83 and P.S. 182 and then go out to the East Harlem parks as well as Jefferson Houses and Washington Houses. The children who attend the program are between 7 and 12 years old. The children were selected to attend the program via a combination of word of mouth, teacher or principal recommendation, or school coordinator. These recommendations are based on the belief of the recommender that a student may benefit or thrive from a program such as this, the child may need structure because of the child's home life, or the child may not be doing well in school. The child must comply with certain guidelines such as being able to walk in a straight line, provide their report card, and need a physician approval to participate in physical activities. The parent completes the application, and the child completes an agreement to comply with the core values of the program (Respect, Responsibility, Unique-ness, Listening, Learning, Energy (Exercise & Eating Healthy), Sharing, Safety, Fun) and that the child agrees to follow instructions. The number of participants in the study for the school year 2012-2013 was 34, and 33 for the school year 2013-2014.

The data collection method used was a daily attendance chart recorded by one of the event coordinators noting when each child attended a program event. The attendance chart is then used to calculate the number of hours a child attended the program per week and the number of calories burned per activity and the number of miles each child biked per week. To record Body Mass Index (BMI) for the children, a school nurse working with Concrete Safaris took the weight and height measurements of each child who participated. This information was recorded on two separate occasions: one recording on 10/24/13 and one recording on 11/10/14. The Public School the child attended recorded the NYC FITNESSGRAM, a BMI percentile twice: one recording for the 2012-2013 school year and another recording for the 2013-2014 school year. FITNESSGRAM is a tool used to measure a student's fitness and is currently used in New York City Public Schools (4). The NYC FITNESSGRAM report summarizes each student's performance on fitness assessments and suggests ways to help the student achieve optimal performance for better health based on their age and sex (4). NYC FITNESSGRAM supports teachers and students (K-12) to effectively set and manage personal and collective fitness goals (4). Parents and children receive results in a personalized report to help develop personal goals (see Figure 5) (4). The Concrete Safaris program also obtained the numbers of days absent and number of days late from the child's school as well as the average grade during the school year.

In addition to the quantitative results, we also obtained qualitative data to assess how effective the program is from the parent's perspective as well and the child's perspective. We asked a series of value-based questions with answers that reflected a combination of written answers, yes or no, and scale-based. The questions were delivered to parents in either English or Spanish. 20 parents and 25 child participants completed the survey.

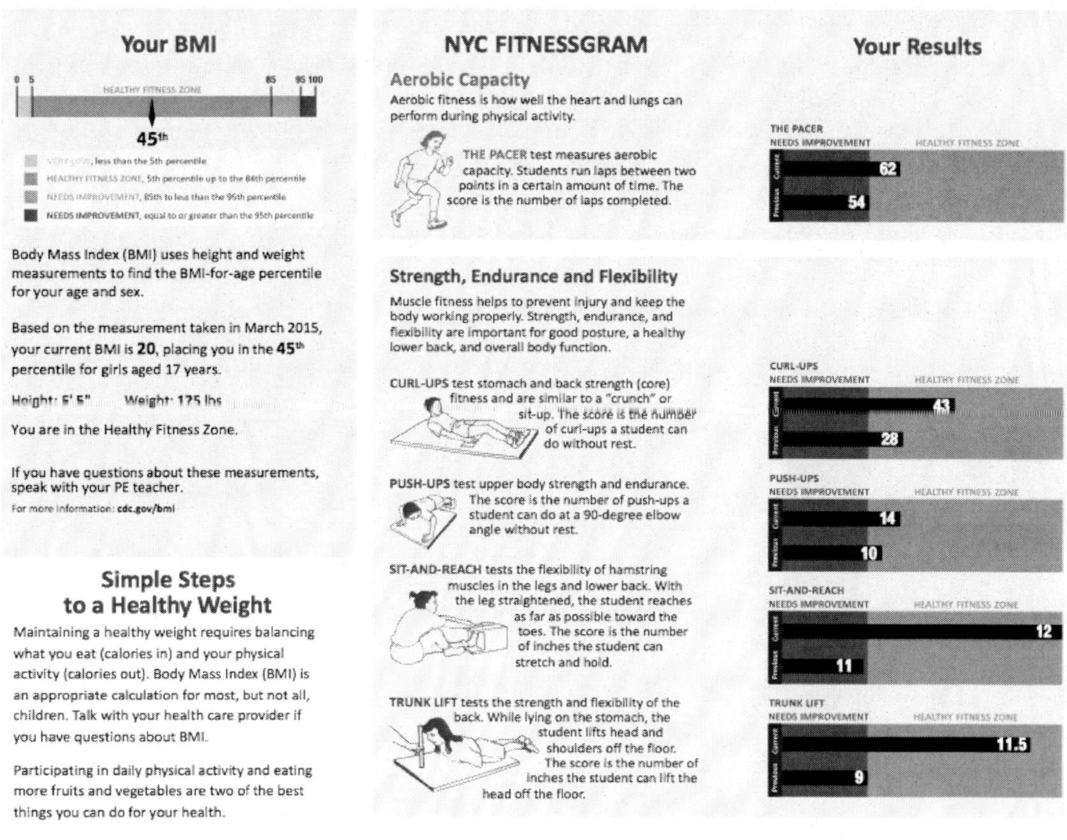

Figure 5. NYC FITNESSGRAMS sample report grade 4-12.

The raw data from the attendance sheet and the child's height and weight were used in calculating the hours for each activity and for each child, miles biked for each child, BMI, and FITNESSGRAM. Public school attendance and grades were obtained from the school district. The data was analyzed to make a one year comparison.

FINDINGS

Phase one results (see Table 1) included the first one year comparison of 5 key variables (Total Participants, High Attenders, Hours of Physical Activity, NYC FITNESSGRAM (BMI percentile), Academic Performance) since the program has been in existence. The year over year comparisons revealed that the total number of participants decreased by one participant. 24% of the 2013-2014 participants returned from the previous year and 73% were new participants. Participants who did not return are known to have dropped out for a variety of reasons: most graduated to a higher (ineligible) grade or were removed from the program due to behavioral issues; a smaller number could not keep up with the program, or the person recommending the child did not fully understand the program and the child was not able to comply.

The number of participants who attended the program over 50% of the available program hours, increased by 50% from the previous year. The NYC FITNESSGRAM statistics showed no measurable change in the BMI or showed very slight changes. Academic performance showed slight improvement with the increase coming mostly from the repeat participants. Academic performance showed a slight improvement in grade point average (GPA) increasing from a 2.70 (2012-2013) out of 4.0 to a 2.94 (2013-2014) out of 4.0. This increase came mostly from repeat participants.

According to the qualitative survey results, overall, both parents and child participants were positive about the impact that the Concrete Safaris program had on the child as well as other family members. Specifically, of the parents who participated in the survey (see table 2), 100% stated that since starting Concrete Safaris they believe their child is making better decisions more often; 55% of the parents who participated in the survey stated that since starting Concrete Safaris their child plays outdoors more often; and 45% of parents who participated in the survey stated their child asks to eat fruits and vegetables more often since starting Concrete Safaris.

Table 1. Year over year comparisons

	2012-2013	**2013-2014**
Total Participants	34	33
High Attenders	16	24
Hours of Physical Activity	4,940	5,678
NYC FITNESSGRAM (BMI Percentile)	70.26	73.79
Academic Performance	2.70	2.94

Table 2. Parent survey

Question 1: What changes have you seen in your child as a result of participation in concrete safaris? Written Answer: "My child is making better decisions more often since starting Concrete Safaris"	100% of parents answered similarly			
	More often	**Same**	**Less often**	**Never**
Question 2: How often does your child ask to play outdoors on weekends or outside of program hours since starting Concrete Safaris?	11	4	-	-
Question 3: How often does your child ask to eat fruits and vegetables since starting Concrete Safaris?	9	5	-	-
Question 4: Is your child making better decisions since starting Concrete Safaris?	**Yes**		**No**	
	20		-	

n = 20. Note: not all parents answered all the questions.

Table 3. Child participant survey

Questions	Answer most often stated:
Question 1: What are the two most important things you have learned from participating in Concrete Safaris? *Answer:*	"eating healthy" is the most important thing I have learned"
Question 2: What do you like about Concrete Safaris?	"I like "biking and gardening" the most about the program"
Question 3: What do you dislike about Concrete Safaris?	"I dislike the "homework time" the most about the program"
Question: How have your decision-making skills changed since you started with Concrete Safaris?	18 stated their decisions making skill were better as it relates to overall decisions, eating health and exercising. 7 stated there was no change in their decision-making.

n = 25.

Table 4. Example of weekly concrete Safaris programming

	Monday	Tuesday	Wednesday	Thursday	Friday
2:20pm-2:45pm	Sign-In/Snack	Sign-in/Snack	Sign-in/Snack	Sign-in/Snack	Sign in/ Snack
2:45pm-3:30pm	Homework/ Gym Free time	Homework/ Gym Free time	Homework/ Gym Free time	Homework/ Gym Free time	Homework/ Gym Free time
3:30pm-4:00pm	Nutrition	Garden Design	Bike	Science Experiments	Weekly Discussion
4:00pm-4:30pm	Community Organize	Garden Management	Bike-Fitness	Public Speaking	Team Building
4:40pm-5:00pm	Community Organize	Landscaping	Bike-Team Building	Arts & Crafts	CS Challenges
5:00pm-5:15pm	Closing/ Dismissal	Closing/ Dismissal	Closing/ Dismissal	Closing/ Dismissal	Closing/ Dismissal

Most of the children participating in the survey (see table 3) stated that since Starting Concrete Safaris "eating healthy" was the most important thing they have learned. They stated that what they liked most about the program is "biking and gardening" and what they disliked most about the program was "homework time". 72% of the children participating in the survey stated that they felt their decision making skills overall and specifically relating to eating healthy and exercising were better.

Discussion

Significant child health disparities exist in the East Harlem community which is not unlike many other low-socioeconomic communities across the nation. These health disparities persist due to a variety of social, environmental and structural risk factors which create challenges for children to make healthy choices that would positively impact their lives. Implementing the Concrete Safaris program, a community-based multi-level intervention, demonstrates that this type of approach can improve a child's fitness and maintain or raise the child's academic performance post-enrollment. The preliminary phase one results of this Concrete Safaris study show a growing enthusiasm in the program. Also, the results are consistent with the expected outcomes the literature review suggests for a multi-level program.

The literature review found significantly more studies of single community-based programs such as community gardens or after-school gardening programs rather than studies of multi-level approach interventions. While there is a benefit to a single intervention approach to reducing child health disparities, evidence suggests that a more impactful way to improve health is to employ a multi-level approach (38). The Concrete Safaris program is one of the few examples of a multi-level intervention aimed at closing childhood health disparities in a low-income community.

The Concrete Safaris program is novel in its multi-level approach. At an individual level, Concrete Safaris partnered with Public School (P.S.) 102 in East Harlem to deliver a 5-day per week after school program to enable children to design gardens, study nutrition and cook. At the community level, Concrete Safaris used the newly acquired land to grow thousands of pounds of produce for the community and created bike routes, designed an annual obstacle race and a carnival. At a public policy level, Concrete Safaris along with its participants worked with the NYC Housing Authority officials to secure land for gardens and testified in favor of bike lanes in their neighborhood. Given the positive year-over-year results, implementation of the second phase of the study will be key to providing evidence of what aspects of the program are most effective in improving healthy food intake, improved fitness, and academic performance in children.

This study has two main limitations. First, the Concrete Safaris program is unique and there are limited opportunities for comparison to other programs. Secondly, Concrete Safaris has been operating for two full school years and has not yet achieved a steady state of operations. There has been staff turnover making the transfer of data difficult and some of the activities have been discontinued from year to year due to a variety of factors including space availability. This has led to some anomalies and variations in the data.

Phase one of this study is focused on assessing the utilization of the program by the participants in the first and second year of the Concrete Safaris program. The data analysis to determine how effective the program is in achieving its goals will come in phase two of the data analysis where a prospective cohort study will be undertaken to assess academic performance, school attendance, and improvement in fitness. The Concrete Safaris students will be compared to a matched control group of students selected from the same school district who are not enrolled in the Concrete Safaris program.

While Concrete Safaris uses community gardening and education as an upstream intervention to impact the downstream effects of health disparities and academic performance, going forward we will also be tracking behavior changes through the school report cards of the participants. From a community perspective, we will also attempt to measure the quality of the neighborhood environment by reviewing crime statistics from the local police precinct. Lastly, sustainability is critical for the intervention to have a lasting impact. We believe the Concrete Safaris intervention will be sustainable through continued buy-in of local and state agencies such as the NYC Housing Authority and the school districts and the continued support and involvement of the local community which will continue to provide the participants with a sense of ownership.

ACKNOWLEDGMENTS

Preparation for this paper was made possible by Dr. Rubin and the Break the Cycle Team.

REFERENCES

[1] Research Portfolio Online Reporting Tools: Health sisparities. National Institutes of Health. Accessed 2015 Mar. URL: http://www.nimhd.nih.gov.

[2] Castro DC, Samuels M, Harman AE. Growing healthy kids: a community garden–based obesity prevention program. Am J Prev Med 2013;44(3S3):S193–9.

[3] Olson EC, Van Wye G, Kerker B, Thorpe L, Frieden TR. Take care East Harlem. NYC Community Health Profiles, second ed. New York: NY City Department Health Mental Hygiene, 2006; 21(42):1-16.

[4] Egger JR, Konty KJ, Bartley KF, Benson L, Bellino D, Kerker B. Childhood obesity is a serious concern in New York City: Higher levels of fitness associated with better academic performance. NYC Vital Signs 2009;8(1):1-4.

[5] Rubin IL, Geller RJ, Nodvin J, Marcus M, Howett M, Merrick J. Break the cycle of environmental health disparities in vulnerable children. Int J Disabil Hum Dev 2012;11(4):301-5.

[6] Kaufman L, Karpati A. Food matters: what Bushwick families' food habits teach us about childhood obesity. New York: NY City Department Health Mental Hygiene, 2007. Accessed 2015 May. URL: http://www.nyc.gov/ html/doh/downloads/pdf/dpho/dpho-foodmatters_brooklyn.pdf.

[7] Gordon C, Ghai N, Purciel M, Talwalkar A, Goodman A. Eating well in Harlem: how available is healthy food? A report from the East and Central Harlem District Public Health Office. New York: NY City Department Health Mental Hygiene, 2007. Accessed 2014 Nov. URL: http://www.nyc.gov/html/doh/downloads/pdf/dpho/dpho-harlem-report2007.pdf.

[8] Anjos T, Altmae S, Emmett P, Tiemeier H, Closa-Monasterolo R, Luque V, et al. Nutrition and neurodevelopment in children: Focus on NUTRIMENTHE project, The NUTRIMENTHE Research Group. Eur J Nutr 2013;52:1825–42.

[9] Smith D, Miles-Richardson S, Dill L, Archie-Booker E. Interventions to improve access to fresh food in vulnerable communities: A review of the literature. Int J Disabil Hum Dev 2013;12(4):409-17.

[10] Hillman CH, Erickson KI, Kramer AF. Be smart, exercise your heart: exercise effects on brain and cognition. Nat Rev Neurosci 2008;9:58–65.

[11] Rasberry CN, Lee SM, Robin L, Laris BA, Russell LA, Coyle KK, et al. The association between school-based physical activity, including physical education, and academic performance: A systematic review of the literature. Prev Med 2011;52(Suppl 1):S10–S20.

[12] Tomporowski PD, Davis CL, Miller PH, Naglieri JA. Exercise and children's intelligence, cognition, and academic achievement. Educ Psychol Rev 2008; 20:111-31.

[13] Greening East Harlem: A community forestry management plan. New York: City of New York Parks Recreation, 2006. Accessed 2015 Jun. URL: http://www. nycgovparks.org/trees/forestry-plans/east-harlem.

[14] Committee on Environmental Health, Tester JM.The built environment: Designing communities to promote physical activity in children. Am Acad Pediatr 2009; 123(6):1591-8.

[15] Galvez MP, McGovern K, Knuff C, Resnick S, Brenner B, Teitelbaum SL, et al. Growing up healthy in East Harlem. Associations between neighborhood resources and physical activity in inner-city minority children. Acad Pediatr 2013;13(1):20-6.

[16] Noyes P, Alberti P, Ghai N. Health behaviors among youth in East and Central Harlem, Bedford-Stuyvesant and Bushwick, and the South Bronx. A neighborhood report from the District Public Health Offices. New York: NY City Department Health Mental Hygiene, 2008. Accessed 2015 Jun. URL: http://www.nyc.gov/ html/doh/downloads/pdf/report/yrbs_report042008.pdf.

[17] World Health Organization. Social determinants of health key concepts. Geneva: WHO, Commission Social Determinants Health Final Report, 2005-2008. Accessed 2015 Aug. URL: http://www.who.int/social_determinants/thecommission/finalreport/en/.

[18] East Harlem open space index. New Yorkers for Parks. The Arthur Ross Center for Parks and Open Spaces, 2012. Accessed 2015 Aug. URL: http://www.ny4P.org.

[19] O'Brien SA, Shoemaker CA. An after school gardening club to promote fruit and vegetable consumption among fourth grade students: The assessment of social cognitive theory constructs. Hort Technol 2006;16(1):24-9.

[20] Libman K. Growing youth growing food: How vegetable gardening influences young people's food consciousness and eating habits. Appl Environ Educ Commun 2007; 6(1):87-95.

[21] Robinson-O'Brien R, Story M, Heim S. Impact of garden-based youth nutrition intervention programs: a review 2009;109(5):273-80.

[22] Ratcliffe MM, Merrigan KA, Rogers BL, Goldberg JP. The effects of school garden experiences on middle school–aged students' knowledge, attitudes, and behaviors associated with vegetable consumption. Health Promot Pract 2011;12(1): 36-43.

[23] Chaufan C, Yeh J, Sigal B.Advancing family health through the garden of eatin': On-site food gardens in early childhood education. Am J Public Health 2015;105:625-8.

[24] Christian MS, El Evans C, Conner M, Ransley JK, Cade, JE. Study protocol: can a school gardening intervention improve children's diets? BMC Public Health 2012;12:304.

[25] Christian MS, Evans CE, Nykjaer C, Hancock N, Cade JE. Evaluation of the impact of a school gardening intervention on children's fruit and vegetable intake: A randomised controlled trial. Int J Behav Nutr Phys Activity 2014;11:99.

[26] Ganann R, Fitzpatrick-Lewis D, Ciliska D, Peirson LJ, Warren RL, Fieldhouse P, et al.Enhancing nutritional environments through access to fruit and vegetables in schools and homes among children and youth: a systematic review. BMC Res Notes 2014;7:422.

[27] Healthy kids. Successful students. Stronger communities. Health and academic achievement. Atlanta, GA: National Center for Chronic Disease Prevention and Health Promotion, Division of Population Health, CDC. Accessed 2015 Aug. URL: http://www.cdc.gov/healthyyouth/health_and_academics/pdf/health-academic-achievement.pdf.

[28] MacLellan D, Taylor J, Wood K. Food intake and academic performance among adolescents. Can J Diet Pract Res 2008;69(3):141–4.

[29] Neumark-Sztainer D, Story M, Dixon LB, Resnick MD, Blum RW. Correlates of inadequate consumption of dairy products among adolescents. J Nutr Educ 1997; 29(1): 12–20.

[30] Neumark-Sztainer D, Story M, Resnick MD, Blum RW. Correlates of inadequate fruit and vegetable consumption among adolescents. Prev Med 1996;25(5):497–505.

[31] Centers for Disease Control and Prevention. Student health and academic achievement. Accessed 2015 Aug. URL: http://www.cdc.gov/ healthyyouth/health_and_academics/index.htm.
[32] Budde H, Voelcker-Rehage C, Pietrayk-Kendziorra S, Ribeiro P, Tidow G. Acute coordinative exercise improves attentional performance in adolescents. Neurosci Lett 2008; 441 (2):219-23.
[33] Dwyer T, Blizzard L, Dean K. Physical activity and performance in children. Nutr Rev 1996;54 (4 Pt 2):S27–S31.
[34] Tuckman BW, Hinkle JS. An experimental study of the physical and psychological effects of aerobic exercise on schoolchildren. Health Psychol 1986;5(3):197–207.
[35] Donnelly JE, Greene JL, Gibson CA, Smith BK, Washburn RA, Sullivan DK, et al. Physical activity across the curriculum (PAAC): a randomized controlled trial to promote physical activity and diminish overweight and obesity in elementary school children. Prev Med 2009;49(4):336–341.
[36] Shephard RJ. Habitual physical activity and academic performance. Nutr Rev 1996;54(4 pt 2):S32–6.
[37] Fedewa AL, Ahn S. The effects of physical activity and physical fitness on hildren's achievement and cognitive outcomes: a meta-analysis. Res Quart Exerc Sport 2011;82(3):521–35.
[38] Frieden TR. A framework for public health action: The Health iImpact pyramid. Am J Public Health 2010;100(4):590-5.
[39] Theory at a glance: A guide for health promotion practice, second ed. Bethesda, MD: US Department Health Human Services, National Institutes Health, 2005. Accessed 2014 May. URL: http://www.sneb.org/ 2014/Theory%20at%20a%20 Glance.pdf.
[40] Strategies to prevent obesity and other chronic diseases. The CDC guide to dtrategies to increase the consumption of fruits and vegetables. Accessed 2014 Jul. URL: http://www.cdc.gov/obesity.
[41] Concrete Safaris. Annual Report, 2013. Accessed 2014 Jul. URL: http://www.concretesafaris.org/en/.

In: Environmental Health Disparities
Editors: I Leslie Rubin and Joav Merrick

ISBN: 978-1-63484-211-2

Chapter 12

PRETERM SURVIVORS: COMMUNITY SUPPORT TO LESSEN HEALTH DISPARITIES

Amelia Dmowska**, Bree Andrews, Michael Schreiber and Michael E Msall
University of Chicago Medicine Comer Children's Hospital, Chicago, Illinois, US
Joseph P Kennedy Jr Research Center on Intellectual and Developmental Disabilities, University of Chicago, Chicago, Illinois, US
Section of Developmental and Behavioral Pediatrics and Illinois LEND, University of Illinois at Chicago, Chicago, Illinois, US

In this chapter we evaluate the impact of accessing quality community interventions in the preschool years and develop an economic model of how access to these services decreases long term special-education costs. Methods: The cohort for this study included 121 very preterm infants who received surfactant replacement and ventilation and were enrolled in a randomized controlled study of nitric oxide for respiratory distress syndrome. These children were prospectively followed to monitor health, growth, and development during the first six years of life. Results: Using our models, for every 100 very low birth weight infants without Early Intervention (EI) or Early Head Start (EHS), the lifetime cost of special education was $13.2 million. For every 100 very low-birth weight infants who do receive comprehensive Early Intervention or Early Head Start services, special education costs decrease by $7.4 million. In order to increase access to comprehensive early intervention early head start and early child education services (EI-EHS-ECE) from 35% to 90%, we calculated that these services would require an investment of $40K per child between birth and kindergarten entry. Conclusion: Our preliminary data demonstrate that children of very low birth weight status benefit from access to comprehensive early intervention, Early Head Start, and preschool early child education services. These services dramatically improve outcomes and reduce disparities and long-term educational costs. Additional studies will need to examine the impact of these interventions on long term physical and behavioral, health and employment outcomes.

* Corresponding author: Amelia Dmowska, 950 E 61st St, Woodlawn, Chicago, IL 60637, United States. E-mail: admowska@uchicago.edu; ameliadmowska@gmail.com.

INTRODUCTION

Over the past three decades, advances in obstetrics and neonatal care have dramatically increased the survival of children born preterm, or <37 weeks of gestation. Currently 95% of infants born late preterm (32-36 weeks gestation), 90% of infants born very preterm (28-31 weeks gestation), and 80% of infants born extremely preterm (<28 weeks) survive (1). Children born very preterm are at high risk for developmental delays. These are defined as the gap between a child's actual development and age appropriate expectations (2). Development is multidimensional and includes physical, cognitive, communicative, social-emotional and adaptive domains. Assessment requires using appropriately normed and culturally valid tools (3). Developmental delays represent a complex interaction between biological and environmental risk factors. Biological risk factors for developmental delay include prematurity, low birth weight, congenital anomalies and neonatal complications such as seizures/encephalopathies, and sepsis/meningitis. Environmental risks include low-quality home environments, harsh or neglectful parenting, parental mental health or substance abuse disorder. Poverty, social disadvantage, and distressed neighborhoods have been repeatedly related to problematic outcomes in communicative, cognitive, and socioemotional domains which are essential to entering kindergarten ready to learn (4, 5). Poverty has also been repeatedly related to adverse outcome in cognitive, academic, and socioemotional performance domains, serving as an overarching risk factor developmental delay and the need for special education services (4, 5).

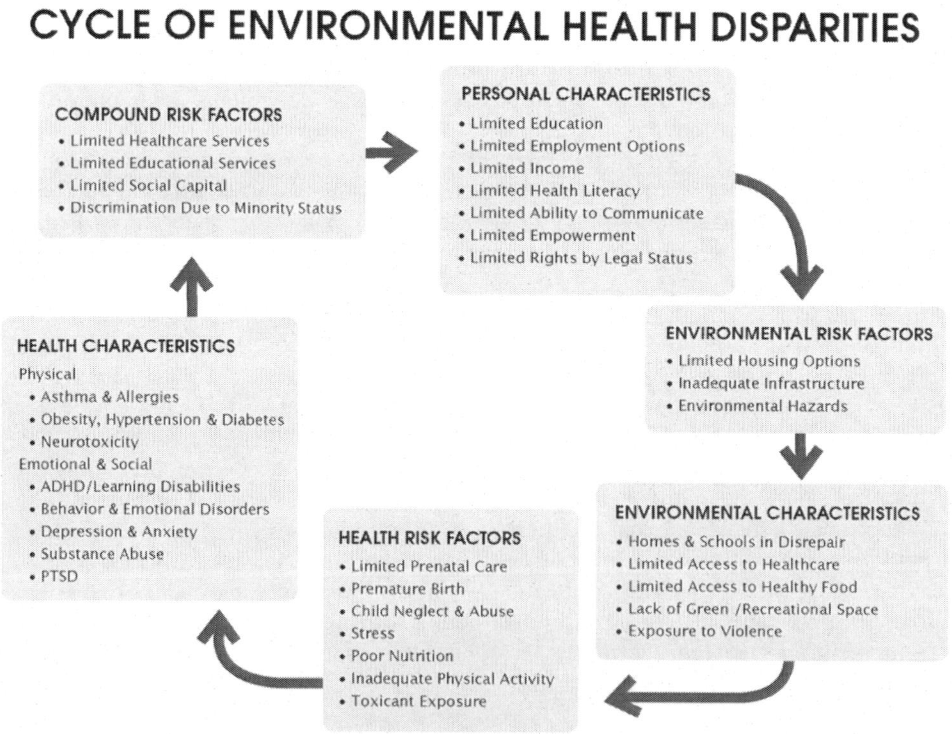

Figure 1. The cycle of environmental health disparities.

Children with prematurity and poverty are doubly vulnerable to risks for developmental problems, as illustrated in the Figure 1, the Cycle of Environmental Health Disparities. Limited parent income, education, and employment opportunities may impact a child's early life and future health risk factors through a cycle of disparity. Research continues to show that fewer children from low-income families (less than half) are ready for school at kindergarten entry, compared to three-quarters of children from families with moderate or high incomes (6). More than 50% of preterm children require special education supports. However, 75% of children born very preterm to families with moderate or high incomes are ready to learn at kindergarten entry. Preschool attendance is one of the strongest factors for school readiness in low income children (6). Attending a high-quality early childhood programs can decrease the achievement gap by reducing the chances of grade repetition and need for special education services of low-birth-weight children (7). Education readiness and early school success can mean the difference between a socially fulfilling, intellectually stimulating, and economically productive life (2).

Early Intervention is based on the premise that identifying children's needs and providing comprehensive quality interventions and family supports optimizes outcomes and decreases future special education services (2). Early Intervention Services include: screening, assessment, referral, and treatment. The Individuals with Disabilities Education Act (IDEA), established the right of children with delays, disabilities, or high biological risk to receive comprehensive early intervention services from birth to 3 Years and preschool services from 3-5 Years and then throughout their schooling (6-21Y). Part C of the Individuals with Disabilities Education Act (IDEA) provides states with federal grants to develop and administer a comprehensive statewide system of early-intervention services for any child under the age of three who has a disability or significant delay in development (2). These services are designed to meet children's needs free of charge, and, to the greatest extent possible, to receive instruction in regular education classrooms alongside nondisabled children and to receive the supports necessary to optimize educational, vocational and life skills outcomes. In some cases, EI actually reduces the occurrence of additional disabling conditions (8).

Intensive mode quality early childhood programs from the 1960s and 1970s included the Perry Preschool Project (9), Head Start and Early Head Start (EHS) (10), Abecedarian Project (11-13), the Infant Health and Development Program (IHDP) (14), and the Chicago Child-Parent Center (CPC) (15,16). These improved educational, health and life-course outcomes for children experiencing poverty, social disadvantage, and minority status (2). They aimed to reduce educational costs by minimizing the future need for special education, maximize the likelihood of independent living in adulthood, and enhance families' capacity to meet their children's needs (2). Evidence shows that high-quality early intervention at young ages, like these, can provide long-term cost savings (2). The IHDP implemented comprehensive home visiting, early intervention, and full day early child education in the first three years of life for children born prematurely. The center-based interventions were created for children with low birth weight, and included 50 hours per week with learning games as part of the core curriculum and college-graduate teachers with a staff ratio of 1:3 (17-20). The program began at neonatal discharge, and all children received medical care as well as serial developmental and social assessments. Children received weekly home visits in the first year and biweekly home visits in the second and third years. The curriculum component included relationship-based learning, communication skills, and parent problem solving strategies for child behavior and family social stressors. 985 infants were recruited for this 8 multicenter study from 1985-1986. 37% weighed 2001-2500 g, 37% weighed 1501-2000 g, and 26% weighed <1501 g (14). These model programs appear to generate benefits far in excess of program costs. However, gaps in quality compromise large scale community implementation and the costs for implementing comprehensive model programs have been deemed too costly.

OUR STUDY

We started with a defined very premature birth cohort as a health risk factor and examined the long term impact on learning, behavioral and emotional competencies underlying school success. We examined the role of access to early intervention and preschool learning experiences and the role of missed opportunities in accessing these services on long term special education costs. We specifically examined what would be the cost of implementing comprehensive early intervention and preschool services on kindergarten readiness and long term special education costs.

Table 1. Social and medical characteristics of cohort

Characteristics	n = 121
Birth Weight (grams)	987 ± 374
Gestational age (weeks)	27.3 ± 2.6
Male, n (%)	57 (47%)
Race/Ethnic Group (Self-Reported)	
• African-American	85 (70%)
• White	21 (17%)
Hollingshead Index of Social Position	
• Levels I-III	51 (42%)
• Levels IV-V	70 (58%)
Neonatal Morbidities	
• Bronchopulmonary Dysplasia	56 (46%)
• Severe IVH/PVL on cranial sonography	20 (17%)

Our cohort included 121 children born <30 weeks gestation who were enrolled in a Randomized Clinical Trial of inhaled nitric oxide for respiratory distress syndrome (21) (see Table 1). All received surfactant and ventilation for Respiratory Distress Syndrome. All had comprehensive neurodevelopmental assessments at ages of 2 and 5.5 y ears old. Adverse outcomes at 2 and 5.5 years were neurosensory disability (cerebral palsy, blindness, or bilateral hearing loss >40 db) and significant delay (Bayley Scales of Infant Development <70 at 2 years or Bracken School Readiness Assessment <70 at 5.5 years). At risk for delay is indicated by Bayley score of 71-85. The characteristics of this cohort are described in Table 1 and included a mean birth weight of<1000 G (i.e., 987 ± 374 g), a mean gestational age of < 28 weeks (i.e., 27.3 ± 2.6 g. Of the survivors, 47% were male and 70% were African American. Social disadvantage was high with 58% experiencing a level 4 or level 5 rating on the Hollingshead Index of Social Position (22). Two neonatal morbidities, bronchopulmonary dysplasia and sonographic cranial brain injury (IVH ¾, PVL, Ventriculomegaly) were present in 46% and 17% of survivors respectively.

Figure 2 describes the overall delay and disability status at ages 2 and 5.5 years. Almost 1 in 3 had a delay or a disability at ages 2 and 5.5 years. Furthermore, Patrianakos-Hoobler et al. demonstrated that 92% of children with disability at age 2 were not school ready at age 5.5 and 50% of children with delay at age 2 were not school ready at age 5.5 years—a greater than threefold relative risk. The comparison group included the 80 children who were normal at age 2 years; only 15% of these children were not ready for kindergarten (21).

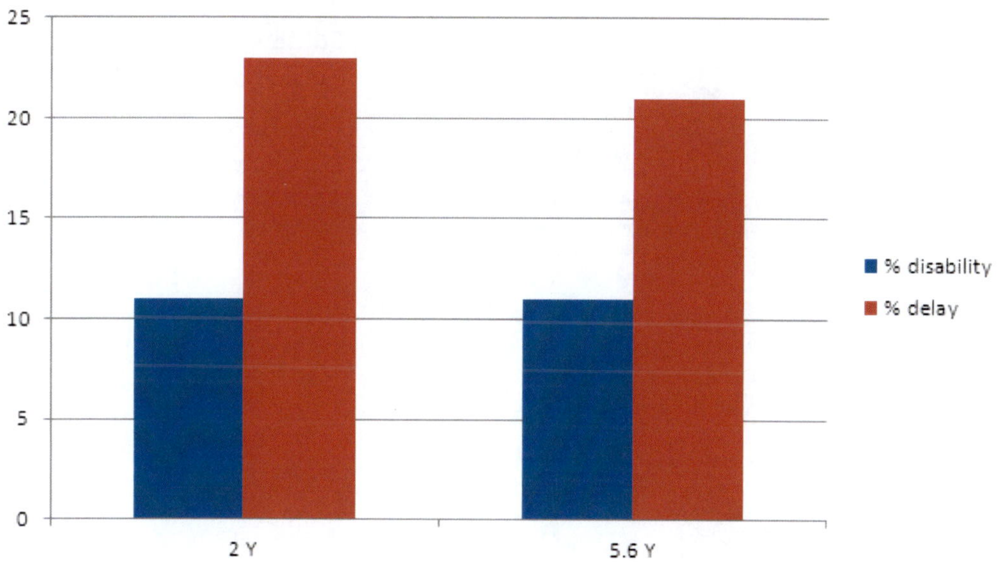

Figure 2. Delay and disability status at 2Y and 5.5 Y (N = 121).

Of note, in Illinois, children with Bayley <70 are eligible for EI but not Bayley scores of 71-85. Among children living in households with limited education and employment skills (Hollingshead ISP level V) and whose performance at age 2 years on the Bayley Scales was classified at risk (i.e., Bayley scores of 71-85) the at risk range at age 2 years, 75% were not ready for kindergarten and required special education resources at kindergarten entry. Among children who had parents with some college and a middle income or skilled professional wage, 7% were not school ready and required special education services if they had Bayley Scores >85 at age 2 year. However, if their parents had not completed high school or were unemployed, more than 25% with initial average Bayley Scores at age 2 years (>85) were not school ready and required special education services (21).

In our cohort, we estimated that 10% of children living in households rated as Hollingshead Level IV or V accessed early intervention services from birth to three years. We also estimated that 25% of children living in households rated Hollingshead level IV/V accessed Head Start from 0-2 years or Early Child Education from 3-5 years. If children received these comprehensive preschool services, then 30% later needed kindergraten special education services. If they did not receive these comprehensive preschool services, then 70% later needed kindergarten special education services. In order to more closely examine the costs of those missed opportunities, the educational costs were calculated using the economic model based on not implementing the NICHD IHDP model. This model includes comprehensive quality services with home visiting, rehabilitation, parent training, social supports and access to early intervention, early child education, headstart, and preschool services (see Figure 3 and 4).

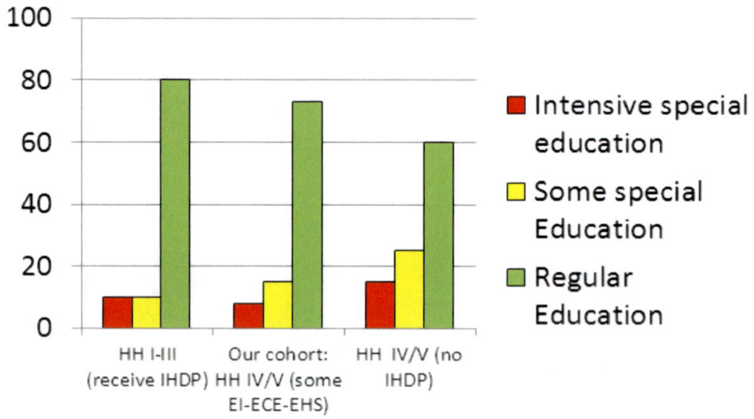

Figure 3. Special education consequences of not receiving IHDP: EI-ECE-EHS.

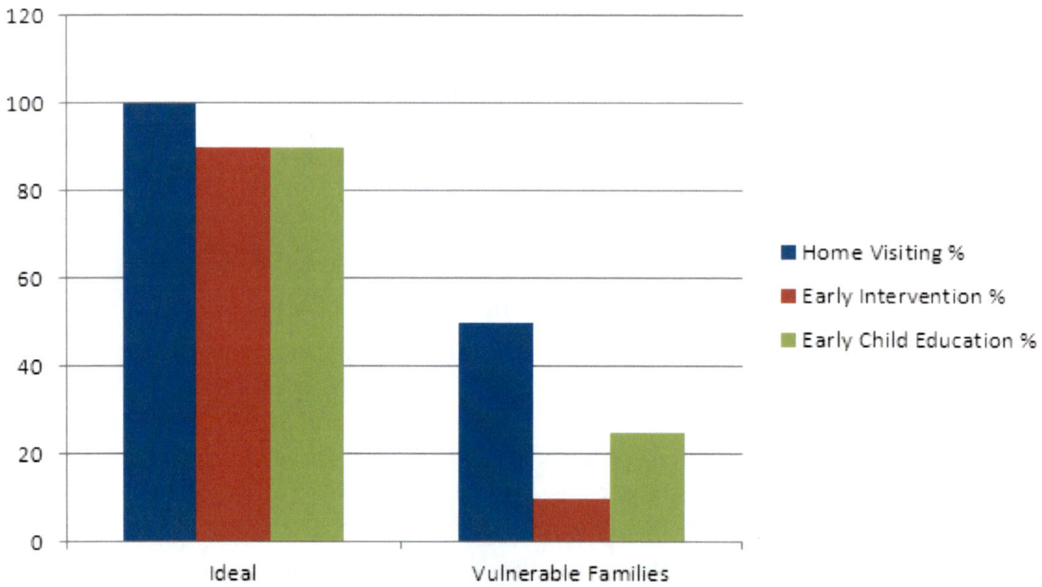

Figure 4. Comprehensive home visiting, early intervention, early child education, and head start services: Gap between ideal and current reality for vulnerable families.

As Figure 3 shows, if children receive the IHDP intervention, then 10% have a disability, reducing the risk of special education services by 10%; 10% are delayed, reducing the risk by 40%; and 80% are in regular education. For children who do not receive these services and have a Hollingshead Level of IV or V, then 15% are placed in intensive special education, 25% received some special education, and 60% are in regular education. In this cohort of 121 children, 72 children were Hollingshead Level IV or V. Of these 72 children, 8% were placed in intensive special education, 15% had some special education supports, and 73% were in regular education. 35% of these children in total received some early intervention-head start or early child education services.

FINDINGS

Using the IHDP model, it can be seen that if children do not receive either early intervention, early childhood education, or Early Head Start (EI-ECE-EHS), then the 25% of these children will require special education services. Based on the Illinois State Department Education Records for the year 2014, the costs for one child per year of special education is $15,000. These children would receive special education from the age of 5 to 21 years, which would amount to $6 million total for 25 children (see Table 2). 15% of these children would be placed in intensive special education which costs $30,000 per year. For 15 children over the course of 16 years, this would amount to $7.2 million dollars. For those who accessed early child education services or early head start, this number is drastically reduced, as only 15% receive special education, reducing the number to $3.5 million for 16 years at $15,000 for 15 children. Only 8% require intensive special education. At $30,000 a year for 16 years for 8 children, this would amount to $3.8 million. In total, the cost for children who did not receive early intervention services would be $13.2 million and the cost for children who did receive early intervention services would be $7.4 million. Receiving early education services, therefore, amounts to a savings of $5.8 million ($13.2-$7.4 million).

A single year of home-visiting, early and comprehensive childhood education and early preschool education in the IHDP program costs $40,000 per child. Only 35% of the children in the cohort accessed Early Intervention, Early Child Care, or Early Head Start. In order to increase this number from 35% to 90%, then this would cost $2.2 million for 55 children total. For every dollar put into early education services, therefore, there is a direct savings of $2.60, as is demonstrated by the division of $5.8 million/$2.2 million. There also exists a multiplier effect because many children with special education will leave school early or require different costly services later in their lifetime, such as mental health services, re-entry to school, or create additional weight on the criminal justice system. It has been estimated that not entering high school doubles the long-term physical, behavioral, and social-health costs of survival.

DISCUSSION

Our cohort demonstrated that children experiencing extreme prematurity and social disadvantage who did not have major neurodevelopmental disability were less ready for kindergarten if they experienced developmental risks (Bayley MDI 78-85). In addition to not receiving early intervention services, these children also had limited access to early head start and early child education services. IN contrast, children in families with higher parental education and employment resources who were able to access both early intervention and quality preschool services had substantially reduced need for special education services.

Thus, there are high special education costs in not receiving early education services after very preterm birth for children born into social and economic disadvantage, as demonstrated by our analysis. Therefore, improving access to early intervention services for infants experiencing social disadvantage and prematurity could potentially lead to significant savings by lessening the burden on future special educational services.

Our model was used for the highest risk preterm infants who represent 10% of the overall rate of prematurity, however, it has been shown that there are additional benefits for 90% of preterm births who were born at 32-36 weeks gestation. These children would also benefit from services but their families experience barriers to accessing home visiting, head start and early childhood education. Additional strategies for auditing home visiting, family supports, and receiving EI and ECE services are needed.

Low socioeconomic status was the primary risk factor for decreased school-readiness in our cohort. Children from a lower socioeconomic status are more likely to grow up in impoverished environments for child development, including decreased stimulation (23), decreased exposure to cognitively stimulating materials (24, 25), and decreased exposure to oral language (23, 26, 27). Although neonatal morbidities impact on determining school readiness, socioeconomic status has a greater effect on school readiness than biomedical risk factors (21).

Table 2. Special education costs for children who do and do not access comprehensive preschool services after prematurity. Formula: cost per year of special education x percentage out of 100 x number of years in special education (from 5-21 years)

Model 1: Special Education costs for Children not Receiving Comprehensive Preschool Services		
Some Special Education	$15,000 x 25 x 16	$6 Million
Intensive Special Education	$30,000 x 15 x 16	$7.2 Million
Total Special Education Cost: $13.2 Million		
Model II: Special Education Costs for Children Receiving Comprehensive Preschool Services		
Some Special Education	$15,000 x 15 x 16	$3.6 Million
Intensive Special Education	$30,000 x 8 x 16	$3.84 Million
Total Special Education Cost: $7.44 Million		
Savings: between Model 1 and Model 2. $13.2 M- $7.4 M = $5.8 Million		

Note: For Hollingshead Levels I-III, some special education costs amount to $15,000 x 10 x 16 = $2.4 Million and intensive special education costs amount to $30,000 x 10 x 16 = $4.8 Million, which amounts to $7.2 Million in total.

In Europe, This was demonstrated by Hille et al. over two decades ago in a follow-up study of 1338 Dutch infants born very preterm or with very low birthweight. At follow-up at age 9 years, it was shown that children from low socioeconomic backgrounds were five times more likely to be in special education (35%) than children from families with high socioeconomic backgrounds (7%) (28). Socioeconomic status and sex may contribute more to school readiness than biological risk factors like very or extremely low birthweight (28).

Early childhood intervention programs may be most effective for children growing up in families from the most social disadvantage (29).

The results of this study indicate the importance and cost savings of providing access to good-quality preschool education programs for children with high biomedical risks of very pre-term or extremely pre-term birth and especially with high social disadvantage. In particular, significant gaps exist in early childhood education services across the state of Illinois, and existing slots in established programs like Early Head Start programs can only serve 4% of children who qualify (30). The Early Care and Education in Illinois Issue Brief recommends that the state prioritize an investment in infant and toddler care by expanding Early Child Education centers in the top ten highest need counties, municipalities, and Chicago community areas. Community areas in Chicago in close proximity to the South Side Woodlawn community area are in particular need, including Englewood, New City, Chicago Lawn, Gage Park, Brighton Park, and South Lawndale (30). These communities, characterized by lower income and employment levels, lack access to services for vulnerable children living in these areas (30) and also have children falling further behind in the schools that they attend. Our data demonstrate that attention to quality preschool education has the potential to substantially reduce special education costs.

There are several strengths of our study. We have a well-defined cohort whereby biomedical and social risk factors were prospectively observed. We systematically assessed developmental states at both 2and 5.5 years so that we would know who was eligible for early intervention or preschool special education. We were able to examine what factors lessened risks for special education and what factors increased risk of special education.

There are several limitations in our study. First, our previous audits had discovered that only 10% of children at highest risk accessed early intervention and 25% accessed Early Head Start. Despite parent permission we were not able to access all attendance records. Instead, we modeled our best estimates of accessing these services. Second, we used previous cost estimates from the comprehensive IHDP intervention - to estimate what costs would be required to implement complementary house visiting, early interventions, and early child education. We could only estimate these costs from available public records. We are however reassured that the IHDP curriculum was modeled after the Abecedarian curriculum and enhanced long term educational and adult outcome.

An additional limitation is that different agencies control data in this process: NICU follow-up, home visiting, Early Intervention and Early Head Start are all in separate agencies. Our data emphasizes the value of comprehensively coordinating these efforts. Our goal for breaking the cycle is to make the ideal scenario in Figure 4 become a reality for children experiencing the double jeopardy of prematurity and social disadvantage.

ACKNOWLEDGMENTS

This study was supported in part by a grant from INO (Dr. Schreiber, Andrews), Illinois LEND (MMsall), and the JP Kennedy Research Center on intellectual and Developmental Disabilities (Msall, Dmowska) and Break the Cycle of PEHSU and ISDD.

REFERENCES

[1] March of Dimes. March of Dimes data book for policy makers. Maternal, infant, and child health in the United States. White Plains, NY: March of Dimes, 2012.

[2] Aron L, Loprest P. Disability and the education system. Future Child 2012;22:97–122.

[3] Smith EL, Nicholson JS, Schatz JN. Preventing early developmental delay. In: Borowski JG, Weaver CM, eds. Prevention: The science and art of promoting healthy child and adolescent development. Baltimore, MD: Paul H Brookes, 2006: 55-81.

[4] Bradley RH, Corwyn RF, McAdoo HP, Coll CG. The home environments of children in the United States part I: variations by age, ethnicity, and poverty status. Child Dev 2001;72:1844-67.

[5] Brooks-Gunn J, Duncan GJ. The effects of poverty on children. Future Child 1997;7:55-71.

[6] Early warning confirmed: A research update on third-grade reading. Baltimore, MD: Annie E Casey Foundation, 2013.

[7] Duncan GJ, Sojourner AJ. Can intensive early childhood intervention programs eliminate income-based cognitive and achievement gaps? J Hum Resour 2013; 48:945-68.

[8] Barnett WS. Effectiveness of early education intervention. Science 2011; 333:975-8.

[9] Schweinhart L, Montie J, Xian Z, Barnett W, Belfield C, Nores M. Lifetime effects: The High/Scope Perry Preschool Study Through Age 40. Ypsilanti: High/Scope Press, 2005.

[10] Ludwig J, Phillips DA. Long-term effects of head start on low-income children. Ann NY Acad Sci 2008;1136:257–68.

[11] Campbell FA et al. Adult outcomes as a function of an early childhood educational program: an Abecedarian Project follow-up. Dev Psychol 2012;48:1033-43.

[12] Ramey CT, Bryant DM, Suarez TM. Early intervention: Why, for whom, how, and what cost? Clin Perinatol 1990;17:47-55.

[13] Ramey CT, Ramey SL. Early intervention and early experience. Am Psychol 1998;53:109-20.

[14] Gross R, Spiker D, Haynes C, eds. Helping low birth weight, premature babies: The Infant Health and Development Program 1997. Stanford, CA: Stanford University Press, 1997.

[15] Reynolds AJ, Temple JA, White BAB, Ou SR, Robertson DL. Age 26 cost-benefit analysis of the child-parent center early education program. Child Dev 2011;82:379–404.

[16] Reynolds AJ, Richardson BA, Hayakawa M, Lease EM, Warner-Richter M, Englund MM, et al. Association of a full-day vs part-day preschool intervention with school readiness, attendance, and parent involvement JAMA 2014;312(20): 2126–34.

[17] The Infant Health and Development Program. Enhancing the outcomes of low-birth-weight, premature infants: A multisite, randomized trial. JAMA 1990;263(22):3035-42.

[18] McCarton CM, Wallace IF, Bennett FC. Early intervention for low-birth-weight premature infants: what can we achieve? Ann Med 1996; 28:221-5.

[19] Ramey CT, Bryant DM, Wasik BH, Sparling JJ, Fendt KH, LaVange LM. Infant Health and Development Program for low birth weight, premature infants: program elements, family participation, and child intelligence. Pediatrics 1992;89:454-65.

[20] McCormick MC, Buka S, Brooks-Gunn J, Salganik M, Mao W. Effect of early educational intervention on younger siblings. Arch Pediatr Adolesc Med 2012;166:891-6.

[21] Patrianakos-Hoobler AI, Msall ME, Huo D, Marks JD, Plesha-Troyke S, Schreiber MD. Predicting school readiness from neurodevelopmental assessments at age 2 years after respiratory distress syndrome in infants born preterm. Dev Med Child Neurol 2010; 52:379-85.

[22] Hollingshead AB. Four factors index of social status. Unpublished working paper. New Haven, CT: Department of Sociology, Yale University, 1975.

[23] Yeung WJ, Linver MR, Brooks-Gunn J. How money matter for young children's development: parental investment and family processes. Chid Dev 2002;73:1861-79.

[24] Brooks-Gunn J, Duncan GJ. The effects of poverty on children. Future Child 1997;7:55-71.

[25] Bradley RH, Corwyn RF, Burchinal M, McAdoo HP, Coll C. The home environments of children in the United States. Part II: relations with behavioral development through age thirteen. Child Dev 2001; 72:1868-86.

[26] Ment LR, Vohr B, Allan W, Katz KH, Schneider KC, Westerveld M, et al. Change in cognitive function over time in very low-birth-weight infants. JAMA 2003; 289(6):705-11.

[27] Ramey CT, Ramey SL. Prevention of intellectual disabilities: Early interventions to improve cognitive development. Prev Med 1998; 27:224-32.

[28] Hille ET, den Ouden AL, Bauer L, van den Oudenrijn C, Brand R, Verloove-Vanhorick SP. School performance at nine years of age in very premature and low birth weight infants: perinatal risk factors and predictors at five years of age. Collaborative Project on Preterm and Small for Gestational Age (POPS) Infants in the Netherlands. J Pediatr 1998;125:426-34.

[29] Patrianakos-Hoober AI, Msall ME, Marks JD, Huo D, Schreiber MD. Risk factors affecting school readiness in premature infants with respiratory distress syndrome. Pediatrics 2009;124:258-67.

[30] O'Donovan M. Early care and education in Illinois: The top 10 counties, municipalities, and Chicago community areas in need of care. Chicago, IL: IFF Public Policy Research, 2011.

SECTION FOUR: WHAT HAVE WE LEARNED?

In: Environmental Health Disparities
Editors: I Leslie Rubin and Joav Merrick
ISBN: 978-1-63484-211-2

Chapter 13

The Learning Experience of "Break the Cycle" Program: Survey of Past Students

***I Leslie Rubin*[1-4,*], *Danielle Oves*[1], *Janice Nodvin*[5], *Robert J Geller*[2,6], *Maeve Howett*[2,7], *Kurt Martinuzzi*[2,8], *Benjamin A Gitterman*[9], *Laura Wells*[1,2] and *Joav Merrick*[10-14]**

[1]Innovative Solutions for Disadvantage and Disability, Atlanta, Georgia, US
[2]Southeast Pediatric Environmental Health Specialty Unit, Emory University, Atlanta, Georgia, US
[3]Department of Pediatrics, Morehouse School of Medicine, Atlanta, Georgia, US
[4]Developmental Pediatric Specialists, Atlanta, Georgia, US
[5]Adult Disability Medical Home, Marietta, Georgia, US
[6]Georgia Poison Center, Grady Health System, Atlanta, Georgia, US
[7]Nell Hodgson Woodruff School of Nursing, Emory University, Atlanta, Georgia, US
[8]Department of Obstetrics and Gynecology, Emory University School of Medicine, Atlanta, Georgia, US
[9]Departments of Pediatrics and Public Health, George Washington University Schools of Medicine and Public Health and Health Services, General and Community Pediatrics, Children's National Medical Center, Washington DC, US
[10]National Institute of Child Health and Human Development, Jerusalem, Israel
[11]Office of the Medical Director, Health Services, Division for Intellectual and Developmental Disabilities, Ministry of Social Affairs and Social Services, Jerusalem, Israel
[12]Division of Pediatrics, Hadassah Hebrew University Medical Center, Mt Scopus Campus, Jerusalem, Israel
[13]Kentucky Children's Hospital, University of Kentucky College of Medicine, Lexington, Kentucky, US
[14]Center for Human Development, School of Public Health, Georgia State University, Atlanta, Georgia, US

[*] Corresponding author: I Leslie Rubin, MD, Associate Professor, Department of Pediatrics, Morehouse School of Medicine and President, Innovative Solutions for Disadvantage and Disability, 750 Hammond Drive, Building 1, Suite 100, Atlanta, GA 30328, United States. E-mail: lrubi01@emory.edu.

"Break the cycle" is a program that uses a relatively simple concept to cultivate the interests of eager students from diverse universities across the USA and from different countries to use their creativity and seize the opportunity to learn the academic skills of research, public presentation and publication, while immersing them in the studies of children's environmental health and children's environmental health disparities. The goal of the program is to promote the students' interest in these subjects at the same time as imbue them with a sense of ownership and potential leadership in changing the world for the better. The track record of students and the diversity of student projects and publications over the years 2005-2011 is a testament to this effort. Furthermore, the analysis of their response to the questionnaire demonstrates the value of their experience and the impact the experience has had on their futures. From the responses of the students to this survey, it can be seen that this is indeed a program with a focus on the promoting health equity for children who grow up in circumstances of social and economic disadvantage and provides a rich yield on its investment.

INTRODUCTION

Break the cycle program is a collaborative interdisciplinary research and training program involving university faculty, who mentor graduate and undergraduate students in academic tracks that focus on the impact of environmental factors on children's health, particularly environmental health disparities. The target populations are communities where the environmental hazards are related to circumstances of social and economic disadvantage. Each student is required to develop a project that focuses on reducing or preventing environmental health related illnesses and disorders of children who live in these communities. At the completion of the project, the students present their studies and their findings at a national conference and are then required to write papers that will be published in a journal. Our budget allows us to provide for travel and lodging for the annual conference and a modest stipend for the student on completion of the project.

Break the Cycle is a joint program of the Southeast Pediatric Environmental Health Specialty Unit (PEHSU) and Innovative Solutions for Disadvantage and Disability (ISDD).

ENVIRONMENTAL HEALTH DISPARITIES

The diagram in Figure 1 represents how adverse social and economic factors may play out in the environment of a child and the impact that these factors have on health, development, education and future for the children in such communities. Substantial evidence, across a variety of academic and public policy areas, supports the relationships and patterns depicted in the diagram. This is the societal challenge of Environmental Health Disparities. There is no question of the need to interrupt and modify this set of relationships in order to change the course to create advantages for the children to break out of the cycle. In the big picture, the task is great and the cost is high. However, that does not mean that we cannot make a difference. We feel that any interruption is positive and can make a big difference for an individual, for a family or for a community. Indeed, the expectation is that the student projects will have a ripple effect not only on the communities, but also on the careers of the students to prepare them to be better leaders and stewards of our collective future.

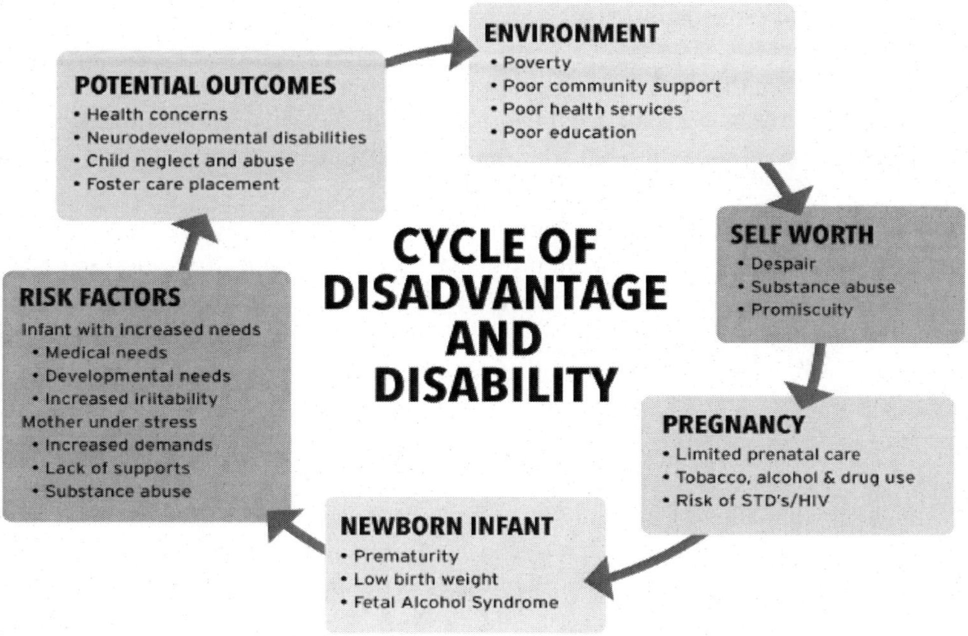

Figure 1. Cycle of disadvantage and disability.

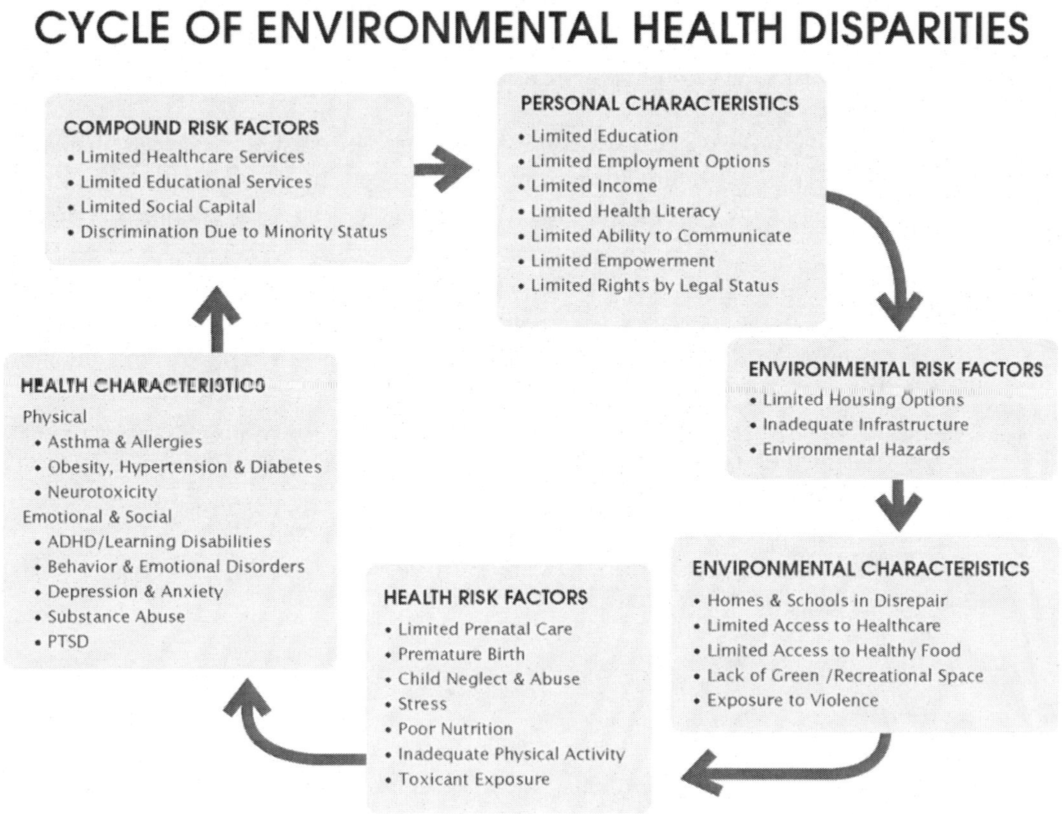

Figure 2. Cycle of environmental health disparities.

Cycle of social and economic disadvantage and disability

We have conceptualized this vexing and complex developmental, educational, social, political and economic challenge as a cycle. The importance of this view is that multifactorial nature of this situation can more easily be approached, and includes the additional dimension of time.

We invite interested students to develop a creative project to "Break the cycle" at any point, and thereby reduce the phenomenon of environmental health disparities and promote optimal health and well-being for children and their families (see Figure 2).

Project details

1. University faculty identify students who have an interest in this topic area, and encourage and support the student in the selection of an idea for research. We are specifically looking for projects that address environmental factors that adversely affect the health of children living in circumstances of social and economic disadvantage.
2. Interested students submit abstracts of the projects which are then reviewed by the "Break the cycle" faculty and 10 of the best projects are selected for each year.
3. During the project period, there are mandatory monthly conference calls with the students and their mentors to monitor the progress of the research projects, share ideas, and help to assure that the project is consistent with the spirit of the "Break the cycle" concept.
4. At the end of the project period, a conference is held in Atlanta, Georgia, where the students have an opportunity to present their projects to their peers and to their mentors, as well as the "Break the cycle" faculty and a a larger academic and public audience.
5. The students are also expected to write papers on their projects, which are submitted for publication in an international health-related journal as a monograph of the "Break the cycle" projects. The papers will also be published as chapters in a book of student "Break the cycle" projects.
6. Funding of travel expense and accommodation to attend the conference is provided for the student and faculty mentor, and modest stipends will be provided to the students at the completion of their work.
7. The progress and careers of the participating students are tracked to evaluate the impact of their participation in the Break the Cycle Program on their academic or professional careers.

The desired outcome

- To have students from a variety of academic disciplines to explore the relationship between adverse social, economic, and environmental factors, and the health and development of children

- To inspire the students to creatively generate strategies to address the challenges
- To collaborate with an interdisciplinary team of academic leaders from different universities and colleges to creatively examine the broader issues of this topic area
- To promote leadership among the students
- To encourage faculty of our university partners to promote academic interest and social awareness in children's environmental health, particularly in Children's Environmental Health Disparities

The questions are then asked, "How have the students found the experience?" "Did they learn anything?" "Has their experience with the "Break the cycle" program changed their lives, and if so, in what way?" "Ultimately, have we been successful in accomplishing what we set out to do?" This project was an attempt to answer these questions.

It should be noted that, although we started with funding in 2004-2005, we did not get funding again until 2007-2008. For 2004-2005, and the first 2007-2008 programs we had funding through ISDD (Innovative Solutions for Disadvantage and Disability, Atlanta, Georgia) and used the cycle of disadvantage and disability (see Figure 1). In the second 2008 program the EPA Region 4 began to fund the program through the Southeast PEHSU and henceforth it became the cycle of environmental health disparities (see Figure 2). Annual funding from the PEHSU grant (with supplemental funding from the Region 4 EPA through the PEHSU) has been consistent ever since. In addition, our current functioning model was not in place for the first 3-4 cycles, so that we did not have the same set of responses to the process. Be that as it may, we have used the data as it came to us for all of the years.

OUR SURVEY

In 2012 we conducted a survey of the students who had participated in the "Break the cycle" (BTC) program to determine what their experience was and how it might have had an impact on their personal and professional lives. At the time we had a track record of students from the inception of the BTC program in 2004-2005 through the 2010-2011 academic year.

We developed a survey through "Survey Monkey", which had a mix of scaled numeric responses and of narrative responses. We felt that the students may have wanted to say something that was not exactly in response to our questions. For the questions requiring a score, the response was calculated on a five point Likert scale, where 1 was the lowest score and 5 the highest. We identified all the students who had participated at any time during the project years and sent them the questionnaire by email. We then reviewed their responses and tabulated them.

FINDINGS

We had identified 48 students who had participated from our first "Break the cycle" program in 2004-2005 through the 2010-2011 program. At that time we were only able to obtain responses from 32 (67%). We did get a 100% response from the students of 2009-2010 and 2010-2011 – both years when we had consolidated our process as described above. We only received responses from less than 50% of those from 2004-2005, May 2008 and September 2009, but interestingly, 100% from March 2008. The students' academic status at the time of their project was: 25% undergraduate, 31% graduate, 31% doctoral, and 9% post graduate. Of all the students who responded, 63% were from Georgia, which is understandable since the program is based in Georgia. 16% were from North Carolina, where we had a good relationship with the Children's Environmental Health Initiative (CEHI) at Duke University, 9% from Florida where we had a relationship with the University of Florida in Jacksonville, two from Louisiana where we had a relationship with the Law School at Tulane and we had one each from Washington DC and one from Michigan.

When asked what motivated them to participate in "Break the cycle" program, the most common responses were: opportunity to present at a conference and publish a paper, opportunity to do as research project, meeting and working with faculty, interest in the topic and opportunity to collaborate with students from different universities and departments in that order; few admitted to being motivated by financial gain (see Table 1). Possible scores ranged from 1 to 5 with 5 signifying "strongly agree."

More than 75% of the students reported that they had heard about the program from their mentors. Others had learned about the program from friends or colleagues, from email, or the internet. The students rated each component of the total experience and reported that they benefitted most from presenting at the conference which scored a 4.58 out of 5, followed by publication of their paper (4.39), mentoring and supervision by faculty (4.32), preparing for presentation (4.32), preparing written paper (4.30), mentoring from "Break the cycle" faculty (3.97), assistance in formulating research project (3.90), interdisciplinary collaboration (3.39) and monthly discussions (3.39) (see Table 2).

Table 1. What motivated you to become involved with the "Break the cycle" program?

Opportunity to present at a conference and publish a paper	4.69
Opportunity to do a research project	4.65
Meeting and working with faculty	4.44
The topic was of interest to you	4.31
Opportunity to collaborate with students from different university departments	3.51
Stipend	2.58
Other (Please Specify)	1.44

Table 2. Please rate the contribution of the following to your experience in the "Break the cycle" process

Presenting at the conference	4.58
Publication of paper in journal or monograph	4.39
Mentoring and supervision from your academic faculty	4.32
Preparing for presentation at the conference	4.32
Preparing the written paper	4.30
Mentoring and supervision from the Break the Cycle faculty	3.97
Assistance in formulating a research project	3.90
Interdisciplinary collaboration in the research process	3.39
Monthly discussions	3.39

Table 3. To what extent did participation in the "Break the cycle" program enhance your appreciation and understanding

The cycle of disadvantage and disability and environmental health disparities	4.57
The complex relationship between social and environmental factors and health	4.47
Opportunity for professional networking and collaboration	4.47
Research skills	4.27
Conference preparation skills	4.27
Academic writing skills	4.20

When asked to what extent the BTC program enhanced their appreciation and understanding of components of the program, they rated the appreciation of the Cycle concept most significantly, followed by the opportunity for professional networking, followed by the complex relationship between social and environmental factors and health. They also appreciated the practical aspects of conference preparation, research skills and academic writing skills (see Table 3). When asked to what extent their experience with BTC influenced decisions around their academic and professional career, 16.7% said very significantly, 36.7% said significantly, 33.3% said somewhat, and 13.3% said minimally. No one said 'none' (see Table 4). When asked whether they are involved in any activities related to their BTC project, a third (33.3%) said none, 3.3% said minimally, another third (33.3%) said somewhat, 20% said significantly, and 10% said very significantly (see Table 5). When asked what they were actively engaged in at the time of the questionnaire, 65.5% said research, 20.7% said professional practice, 17.2% in academic teaching, 13.8% in advocacy, and 10.3% each in business or industry and public office. Of the others, most were still studying in an academic track, while a couple of them were in transition between positions (see Table 6).

When asked about awareness of children's environmental health before their experience with BTC, 50% professed moderate familiarity, 37.5% were minimally aware, while only 12.5% said they were very familiar with the field; none professed to be expert. After the BTC experience, most became very familiar (76.7%), 20% became moderately familiar, and one became an expert (3.3%) (see Table 7). As for awareness of children's environmental health disparities, one was not aware at all about the concept, 15.6% were minimally aware, while more than half (59.4%) were moderately familiar, and 21.9% were very familiar. After the BTC experience, most became very familiar with the concept of children's environmental health disparities, 20% were moderately familiar, and 3.3% noted expertise (see Table 8).

Table 4. To what extent did your participation in the "Break the cycle" program influence decisions around your academic and professional career?

Answer Options	Response Percent	Response Count
Very Significantly	16.70%	5
Significantly	36.70%	11
Somewhat	33.30%	10
Minimally	13.30%	4
None	0.00%	0

Table 5. Are you currently involved in any activities related to your "Break the cycle" project?

Answer Options	Response Percent	Response Count
Very Significantly	10.0%	3
Significantly	20.0%	6
Somewhat	33.3%	10
Slightly	3.3%	1
None	33.3%	10

Table 6. Current activities (if more than one, please choose more than one)

Research	65.50%	19
Professional Practice	20.70%	6
Academic Teaching	17.20%	5
Advocacy	13.80%	4
Business or Industry	10.30%	3
Public Office	10.30%	3
Other (please specify)	31.00%	9

Table 7. Awareness of children's environmental health

	Before	After
Minimally aware	37.5%	0.0%
Moderately familiar	50.0%	20.0%
Very familiar	12.5%	76.7%
Expert	0.0%	3.3%

Table 8. Awareness of children's environmental health disparities

	Before	After
None	3.1%	0.0%
Minimally Aware	15.6%	0.0%
Moderately familiar	59.4%	20.0%
Very Familiar	21.9%	76.7%
Expert	0.0%	3.3%

Table 9. Do you feel that the "Break the cycle" program is a valuable experience for students?

Answer Options	Response Percent	Response Count
Very significantly	76.7%	23
Significantly	16.7%	5
Somewhat	6.7%	2
Slightly	0.0%	0
Not at all	0.0%	0

Table 10. To what extent have you maintained contact with anyone related to your "Break the cycle" project?

Answer Options	Response Percent	Response Count
Very significantly	13.3%	4
Significantly	23.3%	7
Somewhat	33.3%	10
Slightly	13.3%	4
None	16.7%	5

When asked if the experience with BTC was valuable, 76.7% said very significantly, 16.7% said significantly, and only 2 (6.7%) said somewhat. No one said 'none at all' (see Table 9). When asked if they maintained contact with anyone related to the BTC, 33.3% said somewhat, 23,3% said significantly, 13.3% said very significantly, 13.3% said slightly and 16.7% said none (see Table 10).

Table 11 represents selected responses from the students to the question of how they experienced the BTC program and how the BTC program might have affected their professional careers.

DISCUSSION

The most rewarding discovery was the almost unanimous finding that all students rated the BTC experience valuable, most of them (76.7%) 'very significantly' or a number 'significantly' (16.7%) (see Table 9). This question addresses the overall experience that begins with the application process, the selection, the discussion and delineation of the project, the monthly calls to monitor progress, then the preparation for presentation, the travel to and actual attendance at the conference in Atlanta and the presentation followed by the requirement for a written manuscript of the project for publication and then to see the paper in print.

Although this survey had many limitations, it included the students who had been there from the earliest days when we did not have a formal structure. The structure only fell into place after we were consistently funded by the SE PEHSU grant and EPA starting in late 2008, our 3rd "Break the cycle" Program which actually built on the 2nd one earlier in 2008. Over that time, we build a cadre of mentors who would field students for the annual application process. Although the survey only goes through the 2011 set of students, four years and four cycles later (and more than 40 students later), we have a greater track record and greater consistency in the program. To date, we have seven international journals of the student papers and six themed books (1-13). We have presented the program nationally and internationally, and have explored the possibility of replication. We are also exploring the idea of taking one of the projects and getting funding to promote further exploration of that topic or subject and translating it into practice.

Table 11. Please provide us with a brief personal statement on your experience with the project and/or on how the experience has influenced your studies or professional career

- The "Break the cycle" program was an overall success and indelible imprint in my life's journey. This opportunity was a blessing in my life that truly challenged my thought processes. Everyone involved from the students, to the faculty and staff of [Southeast] PEHSU and ISDD...everyone was such an integral part of this experience. In the imminent future, I plan to further her study of eliminating health disparities for all people through the field of public health. Ideally, I would like to further advance the horizons of public health and medicine with the goal of promoting quality, equitable health for all people.
- I believe participating in this project really helped me understand the research methods we learn in class because of the hands on experience. I learned that I am very interested and motivated by mixed methods research (which is the method my project utilized). I also received more job opportunities when interviewers saw this experience in my resume and portfolio. Finally, going to the CDC for the SOPHE conference was life changing for me. I was so encouraged by coming to Atlanta for that meeting that I did a fellowship at the CDC after graduating with my MPH and now have moved on to work at the NIH.
- Participating in a conference where research on the cycle of disadvantage was approached from so many different angles really allowed me to experience on a deeper level the extent to which social, cultural and environmental issues are linked together and are multidimensional. And it takes experts from all corners to come together and formulate the best solution to approaching problems. "Break the cycle" helps students be more prepared and respect future work situations that require individuals from different training and philosophies to work together.
- I participated in the "Break the cycle" project my senior year of college. I am currently a third year medical student at University of North Carolina School of Medicine. Prior to starting medical school, I participated in a year of research. The "Break the cycle" project was beneficial because it gave me more exposure to research that was non-traditional to me. However, it still helped me develop the skills necessary to conduct research and enhance leadership skills. This project was a stepping stone in the advancement in my career in medicine and science.
- The "Break the cycle" conference has allowed me to meet passionate people in the field who strive for health equity. It was an outstanding opportunity to put into practice what I had been learning in my MPH courses. Not only did I learn more about health disparities through the BTC conference, but I also gained knowledge and skills to be a better professional, collaborator, and networker- all which are vital to becoming a successful public health professional. I am thankful for the worthwhile experience and it has helped shape my decision to pursue a PhD in public health.
- I believe "Break the cycle" has greatly shaped my career. I worked on a project about smoking and have carried forward that interest into residency, where I am currently designing a new project in the community health tract focused on the same topic. I also got invaluable research experience and learned that I really enjoy interdisciplinary interactions. Overall, BTC has been one of the most influential experiences I have had and I am very thankful to have been a part of it.
- Participating in the "Break the cycle" conference helped me to develop my future academic and career goals along with my understanding of environmental health disparities. As an undergraduate senior, being part of the BTC conference gave me insight

into the different paths that I could pursue within public health after college. Before the conference, I believed I had to follow the prescribed route of an MPH to enter the public health industry. Yet I was both inspired and encouraged to see the diversity of projects from other BTC participants. These included students of medicine, law, and even architecture. It was especially rewarding for me to be able to present my work to such an esteemed audience as I had begun on this built environment project as a member of the data-collecting field team in 2008. Two years later, I was now presenting and writing a paper based on this very data that had been assembled and categorized by the collective efforts of so many of my CEHI colleagues.

- The "Break the cycle" conference also expanded my understanding of environmental health disparities and how they can evolve into a cycle of disadvantage and disability among vulnerable children. There was such an assortment of research projects at the conference precisely because there are so many different variables that can affect children's health at their various stages of development. Not only was it interesting to see how every project could be incorporated into the cycle, but also how there were so many points at which this cycle could be broken.
- The opportunity to work with a faculty member on an original research project and to present these findings at an academic conference provided me with incredible exposure to the field. Throughout my undergraduate experience, I heard of few if any similar programs and feel incredibly fortunate to have participated in "Break the cycle". Collaborating across universities and disciplines provided an outside-the-classroom exposure to the transdisciplinary and iterative research process required to get at the heart of issues like breaking the cycle of children's environmental health disparities.

As we review the student responses, we find that, although some had found out through the internet or email and some by word of mouth from colleagues or friends, most of them (75%) were introduced to the program by their mentors. Indeed, we have had a number of mentors who have had multiple students come through the program.

To date, we have had students from nine different states in the USA as well as students from Europe, Latin American and from Africa. We have had a number of students, particularly from the schools of public health who have done projects with international populations, particularly in Latin American countries and in China. This international perspective is positive for the program as it provides participating students with another side of life and also the opportunity to have an international connection. Our most recent connection with Africa has been very positive from all sides, and hopefully we will continue in this way. Generally the students did acknowledge appreciation for the opportunity for professional networking and collaboration (see table 3) as well as for a number of students maintain contact with each other after the BTC experience (see table 10). Unfortunately there has not been much follow up of the students nor has there been a consistent strategy to maintain contact and communication. We look forward to identifying mechanisms to do so as we go forward.

It is interesting and gratifying that the reasons they gave for being interested in the program (see Table 1) were consistent with our stated goals to promote academic success and leadership in the students, which are to present at a conference and publish a paper; for some it is a first time. Obviously the program does require a project, which for the students is secondary to the academic rites of passage. They also cite that working with a mentor was a goal for them, as was the secondary (but by no means insignificant) goal of collaborating and interacting with students from other departments and universities. This element is actually a unique one for the students and one that they would be much less likely to experience in any other setting. Although the main focus is on the project, the presentation, and the publication, the awareness of what other students are doing in other areas and the opportunity to interact with them over the course of the program provides a unique experience that endures beyond the actual project and its tangible products.

It is also good to see that their ratings of the benefits of their experience were consistent with their stated goals and that they rated the experiences quite highly (see Table 2). This is a testament to their achievements and to the process, which includes their own mentor and individualized guidance from the BTC team based on the project and the need of the student. They do rate the monthly conference calls relatively low, on par with the 'interdisciplinary collaboration' which is also part of the conference call; but then it is perhaps time-consuming to spend an hour to an hour and half on the conference call when you only have 3-5 minutes for your presentation and discussion, but the monthly calls fulfill many needs. Firstly, our early experience told us that if we did not keep close track on the students some of them would be distracted by other pressing needs and might not be able to bring their projects to completion when due. It also serves to help the student focus the project on environmental heath disparities and shape their thinking towards the complex issues of health disparities simplified in a single diagram. The forum of the conference call also introduces the students to each other and to a different way of looking at the same issue. This process comes to fruition when the students eventually meet each other the evening before the conference in a relaxing reception, where they get to know each other personally and possibly even develop more significant relationships. This is perhaps reflected in Table 10 where they report some degree of continuing connection and relationship. Again, this may also reflect the notion of networking as a representation of the process of social and academic capital that can yield dividends in the future.

Most rewarding and satisfying was the documentation that the students acknowledged increase knowledge and awareness of children's environmental health and children's environmental health disparities (see Tables 7-8). In addition, they clearly reflect that they learned about the cycle of environmental health disparities and the complex relationship between social and environmental factors and health (see Table 3). These particular tables endorse the effectiveness of the program in communicating the importance of the impact of social and economic factors on health, development and success of children. The students also acknowledge the importance of networking and collaboration as discussed above and then they record their appreciation of the practicalities of developing skills in research, conference preparation and academic writing which are the currency of academic success.

Interestingly, most of the students identified as being in academia – 65.5% were involved in research, while a further 17.2% were involved in academic teaching positions. This is not surprising, as we had encountered them in the budding academic years (see Table 6). Another group comprising 20.7% who identified as being in professional practice and a further 10.3% who were in business or industry reflected participation in the open market of services; while 13.8% were involved with advocacy and 10.3% in public office which speaks to a degree of public service which, one could assume, would reflect a commitment to the public good and to help those who are more vulnerable – especially the ones who identify with advocacy. Of the remainder who constituted the 'other' category, almost all reported that they were still studying at one level or another and a couple of them reported being in a transitional stage.

When we asked whether their experience with BTC influenced their academic or professional paths, they acknowledged in the affirmative (see Table 4). More than a third (36.7%) said significantly and 16.7% said very significantly, a further third (33.3%) said somewhat and 13.3% said minimally but none said 'none'. We therefore have to accept that their experience with the BTC program was valuable, beneficial and in some ways guided their futures, which is exactly what we had hoped.

When asked whether they were currently involved in any activities relating to their BTC project a full third (33.3%) said not, one said slightly, another third said somewhat, while 20% said significantly and 10% said very significantly (see Table 5). This is actually quite impressive, because this was one project in their many years at university, so if they were still involved in any way, it is a tribute to the BTC program. We must acknowledge the caveat that they may have been a self-selecting group and were attracted to the BTC program because of their preexisting interests. However, the BTC did give a vehicle for expression and an opportunity to learn critical academic skills, to be immersed in a subject or topic for a period of time to hear about other work being done by other people in the field, and to have a conceptual framework upon which to hang the clinical, academic, professional, support and service related activities.

Table 11 is the exact wording of the students' response to an open ended question of what role the BTC played in their lives. It is encouraging to see how each student perceived the experience and what impact it had on career choices and more importantly on how the students came to think about themselves and their relationship with the world around them. Most importantly, in some of the comments the ideas of responsibility for social and environmental causes came to the fore with hints of future leadership. In a sense, these comments say it all.

CONCLUSION

"Break the cycle" is a program that uses a relatively simple concept to cultivate the interests of eager students from diverse universities across the USA and from different countries to use their creativity and seize the opportunity to learn the academic skills of research, public presentation and publication, while immersing them in the studies of children's environmental health and children's environmental health disparities. The goal of the program is to promote the students' interest in these subjects at the same time as imbue them with a sense of ownership and potential leadership in changing the world for the better. The track record of students and the diversity of student projects and publications is a testament to this effort. Furthermore, the analysis of their response to the questionnaire demonstrates the value of their experience and the impact the experience has had on their futures.

The BTC program is relatively inexpensive, in that the direct costs go primarily towards the coordination of the program and the costs of travel and accommodation for the students to come to Atlanta for the conference. The other costs of the program are absorbed by the responsibilities of one regional grantee of the PEHSU network which is mandated to provide education on children's environmental health to professionals and to the public and cultivate future leaders. The environmental health disparities part of the program is consistent with the mission of ISDD. From the responses of the students, it can be seen that this is indeed a program with a focus on the promoting health equity for children who grow up in circumstances of social and economic disadvantage and provides a rich yield on its investment.

"Break the cycle" will continue its annual process and continue to cultivate the interests of students from around the country and around the world and continue to provide them with the tools to become future leaders and make a positive difference in the world but we need more. While the accumulation of students and student publications is commendable, major problems in the world with environmental pollution continue to affect our children. These show no sign of abating, and the major health disparities continue that rob our societies of the great potential of many of their citizens – both in the USA and around the world, particularly in developing countries in continents such as Latin America, Asia and Africa.

"Break the cycle" is a simple readily reproducible program than can be adopted and adapted to any center, where there is a thirst for knowledge and skills and a desire to make the world a better place. It is our responsibility to leave the world a better place, and what better way to do it than to cultivate our future leaders who will have the knowledge and skills to deal with the challenges of the future?

ACKNOWLEDGMENTS

We are grateful for the collaboration with the National Institute of Child Health and Human Development in Israel, who has collaborated and facilitated the publications of all the papers and books since "Break the cycle" program number III.

The U.S. Environmental Protection Agency (EPA) supports the PEHSU by providing partial funding to ATSDR under Inter-Agency Agreement number DW-75-95877701. Neither EPA nor ATSDR endorse the purchase of any commercial products or services mentioned in PEHSU publications.

DISCLAIMERS

This publication was supported by the cooperative agreement award number 1U61TS000237-02from the Agency for Toxic Substances and Disease Registry (ATSDR). Its contents are the responsibility of the authors and do not necessarily represent the official views of the Agency for Toxic Substances and Disease Registry (ATSDR).

REFERENCES

[1] Rubin IL, Geller RJ, Nodvin J, Ace K, Merrick J. Break the cycle of adverse health and developmental disparities for children. Int J Child Adolesc Health 2009; 2(3); 265-421.

[2] Rubin IL, Ace K, Nodvin J, Geller RJ, Marcus M, Merrick J. Vulnerable children: Break the cycle of environmental health disparities. Int J Child Health Hum Dev 2010; 3(4):357-453.

[3] Rubin IL, Nodvin J, Geller RJ, Marcus M, Merrick J. Vulnerable children: Break the cycle of environmental health disparities. Rev Environ Health 2011;26(3):135-229.

[4] Rubin IL, Geller RJ, Nodvin J, Marcus M, Howell M, Merrick J. Break the cycle of environmental health disparities in vulnerable children. Int J Disabil Hum Dev 2012;11(4):295-409.

[5] Rubin IL, Geller RJ, Nodvin J, Marcus M, Howett M, Merrick J, eds. Break the cycle: Environmental hazards and children. Int J Disabil Hum Dev 2013;12(4):395-478.

[6] Rubin IL, Geller RJ, Nodvin J, Howett M, Gitterman BA, Merrick J, eds. Break the cycle of disadvantage and disability: Environmental factors, education, AIDS and food insecurity. Int J Child Health Hum Dev 2014;7(3): 207-335.

[7] Rubin IL, Geller RJ, Nodvin J, Howett M, Gitterman BA, Merrick J, eds. Break the cycle of disadvantage and disability: The law, health, the environment and international perspectives A birthday tribute to the pediatrician I Leslie Rubin. Int J Child Adolesc Health 2015; 8(4), in press.

[8] Rubin IL, Merrick J, eds. Environmental health: Home school and community. New York: Nova Science, 2013.

[9] Rubin IL, Merrick J, eds. Environmental health disparities in children: Asthma, obesity and food. New York: Nova Science, 2013.

[10] Rubin IL, Merrick J, eds. Child health and human development: Social, economic and environmental factors. New York: Nova Science, 2013.

[11] Rubin IL, Merrick J, eds. Break the cycle of environmental health disparities: Maternal and child health aspects. New York: Nova Science, 2013.

[12] Rubin IL, Merrick J, eds. Environment and hope: Improving health, reducing AIDS and promoting food security in the world. New York: Nova Science, 2014.

[13] Rubin IL, Merrick J, eds. Environmental and public health: Environmental health, law and international perspectives. New York: Nova Science, 2014.

SECTION FIVE: ACKNOWLEDGMENTS

In: Environmental Health Disparities
Editors: I Leslie Rubin and Joav Merrick
ISBN: 978-1-63484-211-2

Chapter 14

ABOUT THE EDITORS

I Leslie Rubin, MD, is President and Founder of the Innovative Solutions for Disadvantage and Disability (ISDD), Research Associate Professor at the Department of Pediatrics, Morehouse School of Medicine, Co-director of the Southeast Pediatric Environmental Health Unit at Emory University, and Medical Director of Developmental Pediatric Specialists, Atlanta, Georgia. He is originally from South Africa, where he trained in pediatrics. He came to the United States to specialize in neonatology and then in developmental pediatrics. He was initially at the hospitals of the Case Western Reserve University in Cleveland Ohio from 1976-1980 and then moved to the Children's Hospital in Boston and the Harvard Medical School from 1980-1994. In July 1994 he moved to Atlanta, Georgia as Director of Developmental Pediatrics at Emory University and as Medical Director of the Marcus Center. Since 1998, he has been involved with the Southeast Pediatric Environmental Health Specialty Unit at Emory University, where he has integrated his understanding of developmental disabilities into the world of environmental health. In May 2004, he founded the Institute for the Study of Disadvantage and Disability (now Innovative Solutions for Disadvantage and Disability), which is dedicated to improving awareness and understanding of the relationship between social and economic disadvantage and disabilities in children. In September 2004, he left Emory University, and joined the faculty of Morehouse School of Medicine. He is the recipeint of the 2012 Calvin J Sia Award from the American Academy of Pediatrics for work on a Medical Home for Homeless Children and also through the ISDD of the 2013 Martin Luther King Jr Award from Emory University Business School and School of Public Health for the work of ISDD in improving the lives of children who grow up in circumstances of social and economic disadvantage. E-mail: lrubi01@emory.edu.

Joav Merrick, MD, MMedSci, DMSc, born and educated in Denmark is professor of pediatrics, child health and human development, Division of Pediatrics, Hadassah Hebrew University Medical Center, Mt Scopus Campus, Jerusalem, Israel and Kentucky Children's Hospital, University of Kentucky, Lexington, Kentucky United States and professor of public health at the Center for Healthy Development, School of Public Health, Georgia State University, Atlanta, United States, the medical director of the Health Services, Division for Intellectual and Developmental Disabilities, Ministry of Social Affairs and Social Services, Jerusalem, the founder and director of the National Institute of Child Health and Human Development in Israel. Numerous publications in the field of pediatrics, child health and human development, rehabilitation, intellectual disability, disability, health, welfare, abuse, advocacy, quality of life and prevention. Received the Peter Sabroe Child Award for outstanding work on behalf of Danish Children in 1985 and the International LEGO-Prize ("The Children's Nobel Prize") for an extraordinary contribution towards improvement in child welfare and well-being in 1987. E-mail: jmerrick@zahav.net.il.

In: Environmental Health Disparities
Editors: I Leslie Rubin and Joav Merrick
ISBN: 978-1-63484-211-2

Chapter 15

ABOUT INNOVATIVE SOLUTIONS FOR DISADVANTAGE AND DISABILITY

In 2004, the Institute for the Study of Disadvantage and Disability (ISDD) was established to address the relationship between social and economic disadvantage and the prevalence of developmental disabilities and to reduce health disparities and the disparity in services available for vulnerable populations. In 2012 the name was changed to Innovative Solutions for Disadvantage and Disability (ISDD) to more accurately reflect the work that had been done and the changing language of this field of endeavor.

The mission of ISDD is to promote health equity among children living in social and economic disadvantage with or at risk for disability. This mission is accomplished thorugh three core programs:

Break the cycle

This program is at the heart of ISDD in that it offers a broad look at the relationship between social or economic disadvantage and developmental disabilities in addition to other chronic medical conditions. ISDD has partnered with the Southeast Pediatric Environmental Health Specialty Unit at Emory University (PEHSU) to expand the concept to include environmental health disparities. Break the cycle is a multidisciplinary academic program that focuses on cultivating future leaders in the fields of medicine, nursing, public health, law, social work, education and other related disciplines. Each year, ISDD invites students and faculty from a variety of colleges and universities to develop projects that will "break the cycle of environmental health disparities" and raise awareness of children's environmental health and environmental healthdisparities. The students present their projects at a national conference and the results are published in international journals. Over the past 10 years "break the cycle" has engaged 93 students from 27 different universities in nine states in the USA as well as students from Latin America, Europe and Africa, that have resulted in the pulication of eight journal supplements. This set of projects forms the basis for this book series.

ISDD was the recipient of the 2013 Martin Luther King Jr. Award from Emory University Goizueta School of Busines and the Rollins School of Public Health for work done in providing health care and other swrvices for vulnerable children and their families.

Healthcare without walls

Healthcare without walls is a comprehensive community-based, medical home model which addresses the health care needs of children who have been homeless. ISDD works in collaboration with Mary Hall Freedom House, the Morehouse School of Medicine, Children's Healthcare of Atlanta, and the Rollins School of Public Health at Emory University to provide a medical home for the children and health literacy training for their mothers. Over 175 mothers with their children have been served to date by this program. This model is being replicated addressing homeless military veterans in the Atlanta area and has expanded to include mental health needs as well as physical health needs. This program is a template for improving the health and well-being of children all over the world, who suffer from a state of homelessness.

Project GRANDD

Project GRANDD is a community-based support program for grandparents in the greater metropolitan Atlanta area, who are raising their grandchildren with disabilities, chronic illness, and behavior or learning difficulties. Project GRANDD provides group educational meetings, monthly support groups, material aid, home visits and individual case management. Project GRANDD has partnered with the Nell Hodgson Woodruff School of Nursing to provide students with the opportunity to do home health visits to the families as part of their training. A significant consequence of this program is that it has resulted in community building among the grandparents, which has promoted a sense of empowerment and independence. To date over 100 grandparents with over 200 grandchildren between them are served by Project GRANDD. This model can be applied to many populations around the world, where grandparents have the responsibility of raising their grandchildren – especially in areas where HIV and violent strife have decimated the adult population of parents.

Contact

I Leslie Rubin, MD
President, Innovative Solutions for Disadvantage and Disability
750 Hammond Drive,
Building 1, Suite 100,
Atlanta, GA 30328, United States
E-mail: lrubi01@emory.edu
Website: www.isdd-home.org
Website: www.pehsu.emory.edu
Website: www.dpsatlanta.org

In: Environmental Health Disparities
Editors: I Leslie Rubin and Joav Merrick
ISBN: 978-1-63484-211-2

Chapter 16

About the Pediatric Environmental Health Specialty Units (PEHSU)

The Pediatric Environmental Health Specialty Units (PEHSU) are an interconnected system of regional centers located throughout North America and internationally, that respond to questions from public health professionals, clinicians, policy makers, and the public about children's environmental health concerns. After fifteen years of programmatic operations, collaborations, and the national desire for protection of children's heath, the PEHSU Program has gained the attention and respect of the pediatric and reproductive environmental medical community and families at risk from exposure to environmental contaminants. The PEHSU program has a critical role in supporting EPA's (Environmental Protection Agency) mission to protect human health and the environment, providing a credible, academic, non-commercial source of health information and clinical expertise regarding environmental toxins and their effects on children.

EPA and ATSDR (Agency for Toxic Substances and Disease Registry) established the PEHSU's to increase the capacity of health care providers to identify and treat environmental-related health conditions, prevent exposure to children and communicate health risks from environmental exposures. The PEHSU Network includes teams of medical specialists (pediatricians, pediatric toxicologists, epidemiologists, educators, nurse practitioners, obstetricians), providing consultation, training, referrals and clinical services to health care providers, governmental agencies and the general public on pediatric environmental health. Medical and public health professionals, as well as governmental organizations, need access to centers of expertise in children's environmental health.

The PEHSU Network helps people and communities with health-related decision-making on important areas of environmental health. The most common five exposures of concern, based on inquiries to the National PEHSU network from 2007 to 2011, were about lead poisoning, fungus or mold, mercury, pesticides, phthalates and bisphenol A. There have also been responses generated around major public health concerns or such as wildfires, oil spills, carbon monoxide, chelation, and other dramatic environmenttal crises like mercury spills, de-icer leaks at airports and industrial pollution in cities and towns. For example, advice when testing for a toxin or chemicals in air, water, and soil might be useful, or recommendations for blood and urine testing.

While Poison Control Centers respond to acute toxic exposures, the PEHSU Network has expertise in longer term, chronic lower dose exposures, group exposures, and what public messages and therapeutic interventions and the development of public messages may be needed. The PEHSU Network partners closely with local, state, and federal agencies and non-profit professional organizations in carrying out this work.

The PEHSU's collaborated with ATSDR and EPA to develop fact sheets targeting clinicians and the public on issues associated with flooding, hurricanes, wildfires, oil spills, formaldehyde, carbon monoxide poisoning, arsenic in foods, medical management of lead exposure, Phthalates and Bispheonal A, melamine and other issues. They have edited books, written articles and conducted programming to give health professionals and the public a better understanding of pediatric environmental medicine and environmental health on topics including:

- School-related hazards
- Indoor air contamination at home
- Adolescent work place exposures
- Hazards of living near toxic waste sites
- Daycare and preschool hazards
- Inquiries about potential toxins, such as residential pesticides, childhood lead, well water contamination
- Environmental health disparities and Environmental Justice

The PEHSU's also provide information via the internet (Website: www.pehsu.net), with a variety of materials, educating professionals in children's environmental health through conferences, presentations and formal university based training programs and working with the media to inform the public about the facts of topics of relevance to environmental health. All PEHSU members serve on boards and committees to advance collaborative activities and community expertise in environmental health issues. The PEHSU's train and mentor medical, toxicology and graduate students and residents from medical and public health schools and provide training opportunities in pediatric environmental medicine and reproductive epidemiology. The PEHSU's have counselled first responders, parents, health officials, and school administrators on how to assess and rectify the damage from spills and other environmental emergencies. They have also provided training to establish PEHSU's in Chile, Argentina, Canada, Mexico and Israel.

The PEHSU's fosters research in children's environmental health and serves to translate research findings into clinical and public health practice. This program is an integral component in the development of healthcare professionals who are better prepared to recognize, treat, and prevent toxic environmental exposures in children.

Southeast PEHSU

The Southeast PEHSU is one of the networks of PEHSU's in North America that serves the southeastern states of the USA: Alabama, North Carolina, South Carolina, Florida, Georgia, Kentucky, Mississippi and Tennessee. The Southeast PEHSU is based in the Department of

Pedaitrics at Emory University in Atlanta and works closely with Region 4 of the US Environmental Protection Agency (EPA) and the Agency for Toxic Substances and Disease Registry (ATSDR) at the Centers for Disease Control and Prevention (CDC). The team includes, Robert Geller, MD, pediatric toxicologist, Leslie Rubin, MD, developmental pediatrician, Maeve Howett, PhD, pediatric nurse practitioner, Kurt Martinuzzi MD, Obstetrician, Claire Coles PhD, psychologist, and Laura Wells LCSW, Social Worker. In addition, Benjamin Gitterman, MD is a pediatrician from Washington DC who works with the Southeast PEHSU on the Break the Cycle projects. The Southeast PEHSU collaborates with the ISDD (Innovative Solutions for Disadvantage and Disability) on the "Break the cycle" Program.

Contact Southeast PEHSU

Robert Geller, Director
Pediatric Environmental Health Specialty Unit
Emory University, Department of Pediatrics
49 Jesse Hill Jr Drive SE, suite 274
Atlanta, GA 30303, United States
Toll free tel: (877) 33 PEHSU or (877) 337-3478
Tel: (404) 727-9428
Fax: (770) 396-1011
E-mail: rgeller@emory.edu
Website: www.pehsu.emory.edu

In: Environmental Health Disparities
Editors: I Leslie Rubin and Joav Merrick ISBN: 978-1-63484-211-2

Chapter 17

About the National Institute of Child Health and Human Development in Israel

The National Institute of Child Health and Human Development (NICHD) in Israel was established in 1998 as a virtual institute under the auspices of the Medical Director, Ministry of Social Affairs and Social Services in order to function as the research arm for the Office of the Medical Director. In 1998 the National Council for Child Health and Pediatrics, Ministry of Health and in 1999 the Director General and Deputy Director General of the Ministry of Health endorsed the establishment of the NICHD.

Mission

The mission of a National Institute for Child Health and Human Development in Israel is to provide an academic focal point for the scholarly interdisciplinary study of child life, health, public health, welfare, disability, rehabilitation, intellectual disability and related aspects of human development. This mission includes research, teaching, clinical work, information and public service activities in the field of child health and human development.

Service and academic activities

Over the years many activities became focused in the south of Israel due to collaboration with various professionals at the Faculty of Health Sciences (FOHS) at the Ben Gurion University of the Negev (BGU). Since 2000 an affiliation with the Zusman Child Development Center at the Pediatric Division of Soroka University Medical Center has resulted in collaboration around the establishment of the Down Syndrome Clinic at that center. In 2002 a full course on "Disability" was established at the Recanati School for Allied Professions in the Community, FOHS, BGU and in 2005 collaboration was started with the Primary Care Unit of the faculty and disability became part of the master of public health course on "Children and society". In the academic year 2005-2006 a one semester course on "Aging with disability" was started as part of the master of science program in gerontology in our collaboration with the Center for Multidisciplinary Research in Aging. In 2010 collaborations with the Division of Pediatrics, Hadassah Hebrew University Medical Center, Jerusalem, Israel around the National Down Syndrome Center and teaching students and residents about intellectual and developmental disabilities as part of their training at this campus.

Research activities

The affiliated staff have over the years published work from projects and research activities in this national and international collaboration. In the year 2000 the International Journal of Adolescent Medicine and Health and in 2005 the International Journal on Disability and Human Development of De Gruyter Publishing House (Berlin and New York) were affiliated with the National Institute of Child Health and Human Development. From 2008 also the International Journal of Child Health and Human Development (Nova Science, New York), the International Journal of Child and Adolescent Health (Nova Science) and the Journal of Pain Management (Nova Science) affiliated and from 2009 the International Public Health Journal (Nova Science) and Journal of Alternative Medicine Research (Nova Science). All peer-reviewed international journals.

National collaborations

Nationally the NICHD works in collaboration with the Faculty of Health Sciences, Ben Gurion University of the Negev; Department of Physical Therapy, Sackler School of Medicine, Tel Aviv University; Autism Center, Assaf HaRofeh Medical Center; National Rett and PKU Centers at Chaim Sheba Medical Center, Tel HaShomer; Department of Physiotherapy, Haifa University; Department of Education, Bar Ilan University, Ramat Gan, Faculty of Social Sciences and Health Sciences; College of Judea and Samaria in Ariel and in 2011 affiliation with Center for Pediatric Chronic Diseases and National Center for Down Syndrome, Department of Pediatrics, Hadassah Hebrew University Medical Center, Mount Scopus Campus, Jerusalem.

International collaborations

Internationally with the Department of Disability and Human Development, College of Applied Health Sciences, University of Illinois at Chicago; Strong Center for Developmental Disabilities, Golisano Children's Hospital at Strong, University of Rochester School of Medicine and Dentistry, New York; Centre on Intellectual Disabilities, University of Albany, New York; Centre for Chronic Disease Prevention and Control, Health Canada, Ottawa; Chandler Medical Center and Children's Hospital, Kentucky Children's Hospital, Section of Adolescent Medicine, University of Kentucky, Lexington; Chronic Disease Prevention and Control Research Center, Baylor College of Medicine, Houston, Texas; Division of Neuroscience, Department of Psychiatry, Columbia University, New York; Institute for the Study of Disadvantage and Disability, Atlanta; Center for Autism and Related Disorders, Department Psychiatry, Children's Hospital Boston, Boston; Department of Paediatrics, Child

Health and Adolescent Medicine, Children's Hospital at Westmead, Westmead, Australia; International Centre for the Study of Occupational and Mental Health, Düsseldorf, Germany; Centre for Advanced Studies in Nursing, Department of General Practice and Primary Care, University of Aberdeen, Aberdeen, United Kingdom; Quality of Life Research Center, Copenhagen, Denmark; Nordic School of Public Health, Gottenburg, Sweden, Scandinavian Institute of Quality of Working Life, Oslo, Norway; The Department of Applied Social Sciences (APSS) of The Hong Kong Polytechnic University Hong Kong.

Targets

Our focus is on research, international collaborations, clinical work, teaching and policy in health, disability and human development and to establish the NICHD as a permanent institute at one of the residential care centers for persons with intellectual disability in Israel in order to conduct model research and together with the four university schools of public health/medicine in Israel establish a national master and doctoral program in disability and human development at the institute to secure the next generation of professionals working in this often non-prestigious/low-status field of work.

Contact

Joav Merrick, MD, MMedSci, DMSc
Professor of Pediatrics, Child Health and Human Development
Medical Director, Health Services,
Division for Intellectual and Developmental Disabilities,
Ministry of Social Affairs and Social Services, POB 1260,
IL-91012 Jerusalem, Israel.
E-mail: jmerrick@zahav.net.il.

In: Environmental Health Disparities
Editors: I Leslie Rubin and Joav Merrick
ISBN: 978-1-63484-211-2

Chapter 18

ABOUT THE BOOK SERIES "PUBLIC HEALTH: PRACTICES, METHODS AND POLICIES"

Public health is a book series with publications from a multidisciplinary group of researchers, practitioners and clinicians for an international professional forum interested in the broad spectrum of public health issues. Books already published:

- Rubin IL, Merrick J, eds. Environment and public health: Environmental health, law and international perspectives. New York: Nova Science, 2014.
- Shek DTL, Siu AMH, Merrick J, eds. Tomorrow's leaders: Service leadership and holistic development in Chinese university students. New York: Nova Science, 2015.
- Siziya S, Mazaba ML, Merrick J, eds. Arbovirus: Public health experience from Zambia. New York: Nova Science, 2015.
- Obeng C, Obeng SG, Merrick J, eds. Health issues in diverse cultures. New York: Nova Science, 2015.
- Friedman BD, Merrick J, eds. Public health, social work and health inequalities. New York: Nova Science, 2015.

Contact

Professor Joav Merrick, MD, MMedSci, DMSc
Medical Director, Health Services
Division for Intellectual and Developmental Disabailities
Ministry of Social Affairs and Social Services
POBox 1260, IL-91012 Jerusalem, Israel
E-mail: jmerrick@zahav.net.il.

SECTION SIX: INDEX

INDEX

C

D

G

H

I

J

K

L

M

Q

R

S

T

U

V

W

Y